T0255869

Lecture Notes of the Institute for Computer Sciences, Social Informatics and Telecommunications Engineering   225

Editorial Board

Ozgur Akan
  Middle East Technical University, Ankara, Turkey
Paolo Bellavista
  University of Bologna, Bologna, Italy
Jiannong Cao
  Hong Kong Polytechnic University, Hong Kong, Hong Kong
Geoffrey Coulson
  Lancaster University, Lancaster, UK
Falko Dressler
  University of Erlangen, Erlangen, Germany
Domenico Ferrari
  Università Cattolica Piacenza, Piacenza, Italy
Mario Gerla
  UCLA, Los Angeles, USA
Hisashi Kobayashi
  Princeton University, Princeton, USA
Sergio Palazzo
  University of Catania, Catania, Italy
Sartaj Sahni
  University of Florida, Florida, USA
Xuemin Sherman Shen
  University of Waterloo, Waterloo, Canada
Mircea Stan
  University of Virginia, Charlottesville, USA
Jia Xiaohua
  City University of Hong Kong, Kowloon, Hong Kong
Albert Y. Zomaya
  University of Sydney, Sydney, Australia

More information about this series at http://www.springer.com/series/8197

Mobyen Uddin Ahmed · Shahina Begum
Jean-Baptiste Fasquel (Eds.)

Internet of Things (IoT) Technologies for HealthCare

4th International Conference, HealthyIoT 2017
Angers, France, October 24–25, 2017
Proceedings

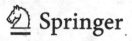
Springer

Editors
Mobyen Uddin Ahmed
Mälardalen University
Västerås
Sweden

Shahina Begum
Mälardalen University
Västerås
Sweden

Jean-Baptiste Fasquel
University of Angers
Angers
France

ISSN 1867-8211   ISSN 1867-822X   (electronic)
Lecture Notes of the Institute for Computer Sciences, Social Informatics
and Telecommunications Engineering
ISBN 978-3-319-76212-8   ISBN 978-3-319-76213-5   (eBook)
https://doi.org/10.1007/978-3-319-76213-5

Library of Congress Control Number: 2018934332

© ICST Institute for Computer Sciences, Social Informatics and Telecommunications Engineering 2018, corrected publication 2018
This work is subject to copyright. All rights are reserved by the Publisher, whether the whole or part of the material is concerned, specifically the rights of translation, reprinting, reuse of illustrations, recitation, broadcasting, reproduction on microfilms or in any other physical way, and transmission or information storage and retrieval, electronic adaptation, computer software, or by similar or dissimilar methodology now known or hereafter developed.
The use of general descriptive names, registered names, trademarks, service marks, etc. in this publication does not imply, even in the absence of a specific statement, that such names are exempt from the relevant protective laws and regulations and therefore free for general use.
The publisher, the authors and the editors are safe to assume that the advice and information in this book are believed to be true and accurate at the date of publication. Neither the publisher nor the authors or the editors give a warranty, express or implied, with respect to the material contained herein or for any errors or omissions that may have been made. The publisher remains neutral with regard to jurisdictional claims in published maps and institutional affiliations.

Printed on acid-free paper

This Springer imprint is published by the registered company Springer International
Publishing AG part of Springer Nature
The registered company address is: Gewerbestrasse 11, 6330 Cham, Switzerland

Preface

The International Conference on IoT Technologies for Health Care (HealthyIoT), is an international conference that focuses on Internet of Things (IoT) technologies for health care. HealthyIoT 2017 was the fourth scientific event in the EAI series and was held during October 24–25 in Angers, France. The conference brings together experts from technological, medical, social, and political domains. The IoT, as a set of existing and emerging technologies, notions, and services, can provide many solutions to the delivery of electronic health care, patient care, and medical data management. The 2017 event brought together technology experts, researchers, professionals from, industry, and international authorities contributing toward the assessment, development, and deployment of health-care solutions based on IoT technologies, standards, and procedures. Thus, it opened a new chapter in the success story of the series of international conferences on HealthyIoT by presenting keynotes, oral presentations, and short poster presentations provided by more than 54 authors from ten countries from various parts of the world.

HealthyIoT 2017 benefitted from the experience and the lessons learned by the Organizing Committees of previous HealthyIoT events, particularly HealthyIoT 2014, HealthyIoT 2015, and HealthyIoT 2016. HealthyIoT 2016 was a stand-alone conference held in Västeås, Sweden, and organized by Mälardalen University, Sweden. HealthyIoT 2014 and HealthyIoT 2015 were co-located events, which took place in Rome, Italy, forming one of the main conferences in the IoT360 Summit. The conferences were organized by CREATE-NET in collaboration with the European Alliance for Innovation in Slovakia, and its partner, the European Alliance for Innovation, in Trento, Italy. Additionally, HealthyIoT 2016 also included the First Workshop on Emerging eHealth through Internet of Things (EHIoT 2016) and HealthyIoT 2015 included the First Workshop on Embedded Sensor Systems for Health Through the Internet of Things (ESS-H IoT 2015) with the aim of using embedded sensor systems in health-monitoring applications considering the future vision of the Internet of Things.

This proceedings volume includes 17 research papers selected out of 23 submissions, with contributions by researchers across Europe and around the world. Among them, 13 oral presentations at the HealthyIoT 2017 conference and four poster presentations. All submissions were carefully and critically reviewed by at least three independent experts from the Program Committee and by international reviewers. The highly selective review process resulted in a 74% acceptance rate, thereby guaranteeing a high scientific level of the accepted and finally published papers. The publication includes manuscripts written and presented by authors from Sweden, Germany, Saudi Arabia, India, Italy, Lebanon, Israel, France, Spain, UK, Bosnia and Herzegovina. A variety of topics are covered including: health-care support for the elderly; real-time monitoring systems; Security, safety, and communication; smart homes and smart caring environments; intelligent data processing and predictive algorithms in eHealth;

emerging eHealth IoT applications; signal processing and analysis; the Smartphone as a healthything; machine learning and deep learning; and cloud computing.

The HealthyIoT 2017 conference would not have been possible without the supporters and sponsors European Alliance for Innovation (EAI), CREATE-NET, Springer, University of Angers, France, the City of Angers, France, Angers Loire Métropole urban community, and other the local sponsors.

The editors are also grateful to the dedicated efforts of the Organizing Committee members and their supporters for carefully and smoothly preparing and running the conference. They especially thank all team members from the University of Angers, France, for their dedication to the event. In conclusion, we would like to once again express our sincere thanks to all the authors and attendees of the conference in Angers, France, and also the authors who contributed to the creation of this HealhthyIoT 2017 publication.

January 2018   Mobyen Uddin Ahmed
                                                              Shahina Begum
                                                          Jean-Baptiste Fasquel

The original version of the book was revised: In an older version of this proceedings volume, there was a mistake in the third editor Name. This has now been corrected. The erratum to this book is available at https://doi.org/10.1007/978-3-319-76213-5_18

Organization

General Chair

Mobyen Uddin Ahmed   Mälardalen University, Sweden

Technical Program Co-chairs

Anne Humeau-Heurtier   University of Angers, France
Antonio J. Jara   University of Applied Sciences Western Switzerland
    (HES-SO), Switzerland
Stefania Montani   DISIT - Computer Science Institute, Italy
Shahina Begum   Mälardalen University, Sweden
Diego Gachet Páez   Universidad Europea de Madrid, Spain
Wasim Raad   King Fahd University of Petroleum and Minerals,
    Saudi Arabia
Titus Zaharia   Télécom SudParis, France
Kuusisto Olli   VTT Technical Research Centre of Finland Ltd.,
    Finland

Sponsorship and Exhibit Chair

Mehdi Lhommeau   University of Angers, France

Workshops Chair

Christian Jeanguillaume   University of Angers, France

Publicity and Social Media Chair

Laurent Autrique   University of Angers, France

Web Chairs

Marie-Françoise Gérard   University of Angers, France
Antoine Jamin   University of Angers, France

Local Chairs

Marie-Françoise Gérard   University of Angers, France
Jean-Baptiste Fasquel   University of Angers, France
Anne Humeau-Heurtier   University of Angers, France

Publications Chairs

Jean-Baptiste Fasquel   University of Angers, France
Shahina Begum   Mälardalen University, Sweden

Panel Chair

Jean-Baptiste Fasquel   University of Angers, France

Advisors

Maria Lindén   Mälardalen University, Sweden
Peter Pharow   Fraunhofer Institute for Digital Media
                                   Technology IDMT, Germany

Conference Manager

Daniel Miske   EAI - European Alliance for Innovation, Slovakia

Contents

Main Track

A Secured Smartphone-Based Architecture for Prolonged Monitoring
of Neurological Gait 3
  Pierre Gard, Lucie Lalanne, Alexandre Ambourg, David Rousseau,
  François Lesueur, and Carole Frindel

Vision-Based Remote Heart Rate Variability Monitoring Using Camera 10
  Hamidur Rahman, Mobyen Uddin Ahmed, and Shahina Begum

How Accurate Are Smartphone Accelerometers to Identify
Intermittent Claudication? 19
  Carole Frindel and David Rousseau

Distributed Multivariate Physiological Signal Analytics for Drivers'
Mental State Monitoring 26
  Shaibal Barua, Mobyen Uddin Ahmed, and Shahina Begum

An Efficient Design of a Machine Learning-Based Elderly Fall Detector 34
  L. P. Nguyen, M. Saleh, and R. Le Bouquin Jeannès

Characterization of Home-Acquired Blood Pressure Time Series Using
Multiscale Entropy for Patients Treated Against Kidney Cancer 42
  Antoine Jamin, Jean-Baptiste Fasquel, Anne Humeau-Heurtier,
  Pierre Abraham, Georges Leftheriotis, and Samir Henni

A Heterogeneous IoT-Based Architecture for Remote Monitoring
of Physiological and Environmental Parameters 48
  Gordana Gardašević, Hossein Fotouhi, Ivan Tomasic,
  Maryam Vahabi, Mats Björkman, and Maria Lindén

An RFID Based Activity of Daily Living for Elderly with Alzheimer's 54
  Muhammad Wasim Raad, Tarek Sheltami,
  Mohamed Abdelmonem Soliman, and Muntadar Alrashed

Automated Recognition and Difficulty Assessment of Boulder Routes 62
  André Ebert, Kyrill Schmid, Chadly Marouane,
  and Claudia Linnhoff-Popien

e-PWV: A Web Application for Assessing Online Carotid-Femoral
Pulse Wave Velocity 69
  Mathieu Collette, Naoures Hassine, Carlo Palombo,
  and Georges Leftheriotis

Automatic Autism Spectrum Disorder Detection Thanks to Eye-Tracking
and Neural Network-Based Approach 75
    Romuald Carette, Federica Cilia, Gilles Dequen, Jerome Bosche,
    Jean-Luc Guerin, and Luc Vandromme

Automatic Detector of Abnormal EEG for Preterm Infants 82
    Nisrine Jrad, Daniel Schang, Pierre Chauvet, Sylvie Nguyen The Tich,
    Bassam Daya, and Marc Gibaud

Non-invasive Analytics Based Smart System for Diabetes Monitoring 88
    M. Saravanan and R. Shubha

Posters Track

Cloud-Based Data Analytics on Human Factor Measurement to Improve
Safer Transport.. 101
    Mobyen Uddin Ahmed, Shahina Begum, Carlos Alberto Catalina,
    Lior Limonad, Bertil Hök, and Gianluca Di Flumeri

Run-Time Assurance for the E-care@home System.................. 107
    Mobyen Uddin Ahmed, Hossein Fotouhi, Uwe Köckemann,
    Maria Lindén, Ivan Tomasic, Nicolas Tsiftes, and Thiemo Voigt

Scalable Framework for Distributed Case-Based Reasoning
for Big Data Analytics... 111
    Shaibal Barua, Shahina Begum, and Mobyen Uddin Ahmed

Deep Learning Based Person Identification Using Facial Images.......... 115
    Hamidur Rahman, Mobyen Uddin Ahmed, and Shahina Begum

Erratum to: Internet of Things (IoT) Technologies for HealthCare........ E1
    Mobyen Uddin Ahmed, Shahina Begum, and Jean-Baptiste Fasquel

Author Index 121

Main Track

Main Track

A Secured Smartphone-Based Architecture for Prolonged Monitoring of Neurological Gait

Pierre Gard[1], Lucie Lalanne[1,2], Alexandre Ambourg[1], David Rousseau[1], François Lesueur[2], and Carole Frindel[1(✉)]

[1] Univ. Lyon, INSA-Lyon, Université Claude Bernard Lyon 1, CNRS, Inserm, CREATIS UMR 5220, U1206, 69621 Lyon, France
carole.frindel@creatis.insa-lyon.fr
[2] Univ. Lyon, INRIA, INSA-Lyon, CITI, 69621 Lyon, France

Abstract. Gait monitoring is one of the most demanding areas in the rapidly growing mobile health field. We developed a smartphone-based architecture (called "NeuroSENS") to improve patient-clinician interaction and to promote the prolonged monitoring of neurological gait by the patients themselves. A particular attention was paid to the security and privacy issues in patient's data transfer, that are assured at three levels in an in-depth defense strategy (data storage, mobile and web apps and data transmission). Although of very wide application, our architecture offers a first application to detect intermittent claudication and gait asymmetry by estimating duty cycle and ratio between odd and even peaks of autocorrelation from vertical accelerometer signal and rotation of the trunk by the fusion of accelerometer, gyroscope and magnetometer signals in 3D. During exercices on volunteers, sensor data were recorded through the presented architecture with different speeds, durations and constrains. Estimated duty cycles, autocorrelation peaks ratios and trunk rotations showed statistically significant difference ($p < 0.05$) with knee brace compared to free walk. In conclusion, the NeuroSENS architecture can be used to detect walking irregularities using a readily available mobile platform that addresses security and privacy issues.

Keywords: Smartphone-based system · Privacy · Security
Mobile health · Inertial sensors · Data collection
Software architecture · Gait analysis

1 Introduction

Neurological disorders are a common cause of gait and balance impairment. Recovery of gait is one of the most desired goals for neurological patients undergoing rehabilitation [1]. Therefore, it is important to have a method to assess the gait of a patient in order to follow its improvement over time. Different methods have been used to analyze gait and balance, including kinematic analysis using

© ICST Institute for Computer Sciences, Social Informatics and Telecommunications Engineering 2018
M. U. Ahmed et al. (Eds.): HealthyIoT 2017, LNICST 225, pp. 3–9, 2018.
https://doi.org/10.1007/978-3-319-76213-5_1

motion cameras [2], endurance using specialized treadmills [3], or walkways with different types of sensors [4]. However, these approaches require highly specialized and costly equipment in a specific location. An alternative rely on the use of common walking tests – e.g. Dynamic Gait Index (DGI) and Functional Gait Assessment (FGA) – that were developed to capture walking problems in maintaining stability during gait activities and determine falls risk. These tests are conducted in a visual manner by physical therapists, so they provide qualitative results and may be subject to some errors compared to tests that collect data. Recently, mobile health has proven to be a useful tool in health monitoring [5] and has spurred the development of mobile systems capable of collecting quantitative data on gait [6–10].

Most of the existing mobile systems collect and transmit sensor data to a remote site such as a hospital server for clinical analysis. Data transmission is done over the Internet, where mobile telecommunication standards such as 4G allow continuous monitoring even when the patient is outside the home. However, what is often forgotten is that these data are related to a person and are vulnerable when transmitted over the Internet. They can be used to model and even digitally clone the person. In this context, one important issue is how to effectively collect and manage personal data with sufficient security protection [11]. Currently, very few works addresses the issue of privacy and security of the personal data. In this work, we developed a smartphone-based architecture for prolonged monitoring and proposed some preliminary routes in terms of privacy and security of the personal data. Although of very wide application,

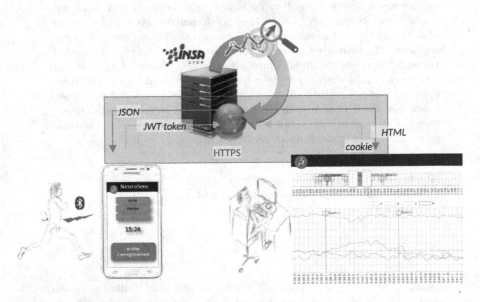

Fig. 1. Overall system architecture and communication. Communication protocols and formats are displayed in green and authentication security tools in orange. (Color figure online)

NeuroSENS offers a first application to evaluate patient's gait and detect intermittent claudication and gait asymmetry. This detection is performed from the duty cycle and autocorrelation peaks ratios of the vertical accelerometer signal and from the patient's trunk rotation estimated by the fusion of accelerometer, gyroscope and magnetometer signals in 3D.

2 Motivation and Objectives

Our work focuses on patient-centered design to develop a technology that is accessible, ergonomic and secured. Building the system around its users helps to provide a sustainable structure accepted by the patients and simplicity to the end-users. NeuroSENS is a smartphone-based architecture that utilizes the sensors of the smartphone to collect data on gait, and utilize computing performance and storage of a server to monitor gait evolution in time. Figure 1 displays the overall system architecture and data flow. The system consists in three parts. The first part (see Fig. 1-left) is a mobile app for sensor data collection on patient's gait and interaction with the patient. The second part (see Fig. 1-middle) consists in a server and associated services to process the sensor data and stores the results on a database. And the third part (see Fig. 1-right) is a client service for viewing data by the patient and the clinician. The mobile and web apps respectively communicate with the server using the HTTP protocol and the JSON format to transmit the data.

3 Architecture

To ensure a good level of privacy and security to the end-users, we decided to set up an in-depth defense system, which consists in using at each layer of our system (see Fig. 2) specific security techniques to limit the damages of a possible attack.

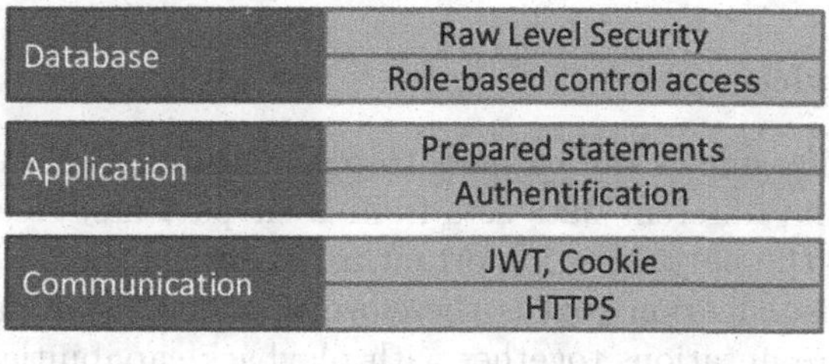

Database	Raw Level Security
	Role-based control access
Application	Prepared statements
	Authentification
Communication	JWT, Cookie
	HTTPS

Fig. 2. Defence-in-depth strategy of the architecture

3.1 Mobile App

The goal of the mobile app is to enable the patient to configure a deployment (choice of sensors and tests) and capture data. The mobile app generates its own triggers to transfer the sensor data. Two criteria are taken into account: Wi-Fi needs to be available and battery level has to be greater than 20%. If these two criteria are satisfied, the time-stamped raw data are temporarily stored until they reach a desired data packet size and then are transferred to the server and the database. A default mode was conceived to ensure that the data will be sent at least once a day (even if there is no generated trigger). Data are securely transmitted between mobile app and server using JSON Web Token (JWT) and HyperText Transfer Protocol Secure (HTTPS). This information can be verified and trusted because it is digitally signed. In our case, JWTs are signed using a keyed-hash message authentication code (HMAC) and allow to identify a device hence a user.

3.2 Server and Associated Services

The server accepts packet transfer of patient data from the mobile app. The data are stored into a relational database, where they are separated into two databases: a research database that consists of all the sensor data, saved as they were received and a key database that consists of the identifiers for mobile and web apps (see cookies and JWT in the following). To enforce data security, the database has a role-based access control (RBAC) policy where the access decisions are based on the roles that users have. Clinicians and patients will not have the same rights in the database. For example, a clinician can insert a patient but cannot insert data whereas a patient can only insert data. Below this layer, we added a row-level security, that enables to control access to rows of the database table based on the characteristics of the user executing a query (e.g., patient has only access to his data). The server also acts as a data analysis agent that supplies gait parameters.

3.3 Client Service

The web application allows the patients to see their different data-sets and the clinicians to see the different data-sets from their patients. Access to raw and processed data by the patients is important to encourage them to become active participants. A visualization tool is therefore provided in an easy to manipulate graphical representations together with playback capabilities: (i) for all the measurements taken by the patient (appearing in the form of a dated list) the visualization is carried out in relation to the events specified by the user during the acquisition or detected automatically by the signal processing, (ii) the user can then decide to focus on an event to visualize the raw signals and the indicators given by the signal processing. Data are securely transmitted between web app and server using secure cookies and HTTPS. Session cookies allow the web app to identify and memorize a user and hence to browse the pages of the web app without having to re-identify each time. The user automatically connects to the database from this point on. So individuals who do not have login/password cannot do/see anything because they cannot authenticate themselves to connect to the database. Above this layer, we developed prepared statements to avoid SQL injections into the database when accessing user data.

4   Implementation

Our mobile app was developed for devices running Android 5.0 as a minimum. It uses the Android Sensor API to communicate with the sensors of the mobile phone and the Volley library to transmit network data. The server uses Node.js – a software platform in JavaScript oriented to network applications – and hosts a PostgreSQL relational database for storing sensor data and runs Java algorithms for processing and analyzing data stored in the database. The web application is mainly developed in Javascript. Jade, CSS and various Jade-Boostrap models are used respectively for the application interface, style and visual application. Finally, the Chart.js library allows us to create animated graphics in our web application.

5   Signal Processing and Evaluation

For this study, the patient's smartphone has been fixed at the waist by a fastening system for the sport. Data from the accelerometer, gyroscope and magnetometer sensors are merged and processed. Autocorrelation of the accelerometer signal along the vertical axis is used to detect the steps and segment them automatically. The ratio between odd and even peaks of autocorrelation are computed to quantify the symmetry of the gait. An adaptative threshold on the signal of the accelerometer along the vertical axis is applied to binarize the signal between support phase (0) and oscillating phase (1) and then computing the corresponding duty cycle to quantify fatigue in walking [12]. The fusion of data from the accelerometer, gyroscope and magnetometer (Android API Rotation Vector) enables to detect the rotation of the trunk around the vertical axis which makes it possible to know the orientation of the step in the horizontal plane and therefore to detect a deviation (mean and cumulative, in cm) with respect to the straight path and differentiating left step (positive angle) and right step (negative angle).

The system was tested and evaluated by recruiting volunteers to use this system. The study instructions were given to volunteers and explained by the principal investigator. We recruited 40 volunteers for exercises on a treadmill involving different speeds (1, 2 and 4 km/h), durations (2, 4 and 10 min) and constrains (free walk or use of knee brace). All the sensor data were collected through the presented mobile app. We validated duty cycles, autocorrelation peaks ratio extracted from the sensor data by comparing them with the acquisition of images made laterally to the patient with a high frame rate video camera (Gige Vision). Estimated duty cycles, autocorrelation peaks ratios and trunk rotations showed statistically significant difference ($p < 0.05$) with knee brace compared to free walk. This is more pronounced as the duration and the speed during acquisition are high: $p = 0.04$ with speed $= 1\,$km/h and duration $= 2\,$min versus $p = 0.009$ with speed $= 4\,$km/h and duration $= 10\,$min.

6 Conclusion

There is a rapid increase in health-related applications. This is why research on these applications is important. To conduct it effectively, the system architecture must protect privacy, provide security measures and improve accessibility for all actors, including researchers. In this study, we designed a secured smartphone-based system, NeuroSENS, for prolonged monitoring of neurological gait. It is made accessible online at http://neurosens.creatis.insa-lyon.fr. This work proposes some preliminary routes in terms of privacy and security for the personal data by a three levels defense-in-depth strategy: at the data storage level, the mobile and web apps level and the data transmission level. This system could be extended to assessment of other walking irregularities.

References

1. Veerbeek, J.M., van Wegen, E., van Peppen, R., et al.: What is the evidence for physical therapy poststroke? a systematic review and meta-analysis. PLoS ONE 9(2), e87987 (2014)
2. Pfister, A., West, A.M., Bronner, S., Noah, J.A.: Comparative abilities of Microsoft Kinect and Vicon 3D motion capture for gait analysis. J. Med. Eng. Technol. 38(5), 274–280 (2014)
3. Kalron, A.: Association between perceived fatigue and gait parameters measured by an instrumented treadmill in people with multiple sclerosis: a cross-sectional study. J. NeuroEng. Rehabil. 12(1), 34 (2015)
4. Rasch, A., Dalén, N., Berg, H.E.: Muscle strength, gait, and balance in 20 patients with hip osteoarthritis followed for 2 years after THA. Acta Orthopaedica 81(2), 183–188 (2010)
5. Patel, S., Park, H., Bonato, P., Chan, L., Rodgers, M.: A review of wearable sensors and systems with application in rehabilitation. J. NeuroEng. Rehabil. 9(1), 1–17 (2012)
6. Fontecha, J., Hervás, R., Bravo, J., Navarro, F.J.: A mobile and ubiquitous approach for supporting frailty assessment in elderly people. J. Med. Internet Res. 15(9), e197 (2013)
7. Pan, D., Dhall, R., Lieberman, A., Petitti, D.B.: A mobile cloud-based parkinson's disease assessment system for home-based monitoring. JMIR mHealth uHealth 3(1), e29 (2015)
8. Capecci, M., Pepa, L., Verdini, F., Ceravolo, M.G.: A smartphone-based architecture to detect and quantify freezing of gait in Parkinson's disease. Gait Posture 50, 28–33 (2016)
9. Weiss, G.M., Lockhart, J.W., Pulickal, T.T., et al.: Actitracker: a smartphone-based activity recognition system for improving health and well-being. In: IEEE Data Science and Advanced Analytics (DSAA) International Conference (2016)

10. Perez, A.A., Labrador, M.A.: A smartphone-based system for clinical gait assessment. In: IEEE Smart Computing (SMARTCOMP) International Conference (2016)
11. Kotz, D., Gunter, C.A., Kumar, S., Weiner, J.P.: Privacy and security in mobile health: a research agenda. Computer 49(6), 22–30 (2016)
12. Frindel, C., Rousseau, D.: How accurate are smartphone accelerometers to identify intermittent claudication? In: International Conference on IoT Technologies for HealthCare (2017)

Vision-Based Remote Heart Rate Variability Monitoring Using Camera

Hamidur Rahman[⊠], Mobyen Uddin Ahmed, and Shahina Begum

School of Innovation, Design and Engineering,
Mälardalen University, 72123 Västerås, Sweden
{hamidur.rahman, mobyenuddin.ahmed,
shahina.begum}@mdh.se

Abstract. Heart Rate Variability (HRV) is one of the important physiological parameter which is used to early detect many fatal disease. In this paper a non-contact remote Heart Rate Variability (HRV) monitoring system is developed using the facial video based on color variation of facial skin caused by cardiac pulse. The lab color space of the facial video is used to extract color values of skin and signal processing algorithms i.e., Fast Fourier Transform (FFT), Independent Component Analysis (ICA), Principle Component Analysis (PCA) are applied to monitor HRV. First, R peak is detected from the color variation of skin and then Inter-Beat-Interval (IBI) is calculated for every consecutive R-R peak. HRV features are then calculated based on IBI both in time and frequency domain. MySQL and PHP programming language is used to store, monitor and display HRV parameters remotely. In this study, HRV is quantified and compared with a reference measurement where a high degree of similarities is achieved. This technology has significant potential for advancing personal health care especially for telemedicine.

Keywords: Physiological signals · Heart rate · Inter-beat-interval
Heart-rate-variability · Non-contact · Remote monitoring

1 Introduction

Remote health monitoring is an important topic by the research community and growing so fast [20, 21]. Here, most of the systems are developed using sensors that is attached with patients [22, 23]. However, non-contact based physiological parameters monitoring using camera is limited and one of the pioneer and advanced technology today. Recently, non-contact system have been developed both in offline and real time using different color space such as RGB [1], Lab [2], YCbCr [3] etc. This kind of technology is not attached with the body and therefore it is completely electrical interference free.

HRV is one of the important physiological parameters which is calculated from the variation of time interval between two consecutive heart beats. Many fatal diseases can be detected early using the HRV measurement, i.e. HRV is used to detect mortality after myocardial infarction [4]. HRV is related to acute myocardial infarction which can be detected from mean HR [5]. HRV is also useful to estimate stress level, cognitive

© ICST Institute for Computer Sciences, Social Informatics and Telecommunications Engineering 2018
M. U. Ahmed et al. (Eds.): HealthyIoT 2017, LNICST 225, pp. 10–18, 2018.
https://doi.org/10.1007/978-3-319-76213-5_2

load, pain etc. For example, HRV features are used to estimate cognitive performance of workers [6] and stress level has been estimated using facial video in [7]. There are several approaches to calculate HRV such as [8–11] where RGB color space is used to extract color variation of facial skin. A number of HRV features both in time domain and frequency domain have been extracted using smart phone PPG [12]. Other methods such as adaptive facial regions [13] and pupillary fluctuations are used to calculate HRV features [14]. In 2014, Xiaobi et al. have used Normalized Mean Least Square (NLMS) adaptive filter to reduce environmental illumination from RGB facial images to calculate HR and HRV [15]. NMLS filter is very sensitive to the scaling of the input light source and the calculation is also very complex. Another method has been proposed by Zhang et al. to eliminate environmental illuminance during real time HR monitoring using YCbCr images of the facial skin [3]. Most of the remote monitoring technologies use the word 'remote' in abstract form which means monitoring physiological parameters from 0.5–1 m away from test subject [9, 15–17].

This paper presents a non-contact remote monitoring system of HRV based on Lab color space using a web camera. Even though our intention is to estimate HRV for stress management, but only HRV features estimation are limited in this article. Here, three signal processing algorithms (FFT, ICA and PCA) have been applied on the color channels to detect R-peaks from where HR, IBI and HRV are extracted. 1st HR is calculated from R-peaks and IBI is calculated from all consecutive R-R intervals in a certain time length. Subsequently, both the time domain and the frequency domain HRV features are calculated based on IBI. A reference sensor system called cStress[1] is used to quantify the proposed system.

The rest of the paper is organized as follows: Sect. 2 describes materials and methods including data collection procedures, feature extraction, approach color signal processing, and Sect. 3 presents results and evaluation. Finally, Sect. 4 summarizes the work.

2 Materials and Methods

2.1 Data Collection

Data acquisition is conducted on 10 participants (all are Male) of different ages (25 to 50 years) and the participants have different skin colors. The ethnicity of two participants is European, other two are Arabian and the rest six are from south Asian. The experiments have been conducted in a Lab in normal sitting position where there is a varying amount of ambient sunlight and artificial electrical light. All the participants signed a letter of consent and they are informed about the aim of the study. They sit on a chair in front of a laptop computer at a distance of approximately 0.5 m and they are allowed to move their hands and body. A built-in webcam (HP HD webcam) is used to record the facial video of the test participants for five minutes and all the videos are

---

[1] http://stressmedicin.se/neuro-psykofysilogiska-matsystem/cstress-matsystem/.

saved in a local computer in .avi format. During the experiment, the average frame rate of the camera was 12 frames per second (fps). First, RGB color values of facial skin are extracted and then it is converted into Lab color space [2]. All these raw color values are uploaded in the cloud server into MySQL database using MATLAB R2017a. Then HR, IBI and HRV features are calculated based on the raw signals and stored them again into MySQL database in the cloud sever. Simultaneously, HR and IBI are also recorded using cStress system with a sampling frequency of 4 Hz and saved in a excel file in the local computer which are then transferred into a cloud server in MySQL database.

2.2   Methods

A non-contact based HRV features monitoring system is developed to monitor patient remotely. Here, a patient can sit in front of a camera at his/her home and doctor can see his/her HRV from a distance place.

Even though, in this small study, both the uploading and downloading activities have been conducted in a local computer but these activities can be done using e.g., Wired/Wireless, VSAT, GPS connection and similarly it can be displayed in e.g., mobile phone, laptop, ipad or any other display using any of the above connection. First both the raw data of the camera and sensor are sent to cloud server using Matlab R2017a. The raw data of the camera is an average color values of Lab color space are extracted from ROI for every frame with a sampling frequency of 12 Hz. From the reference sensor system, HR and IBI are recorded directly where sampling frequency is 4 Hz. For HRV feature calculation, a Matlab script is running as a service in the cloud which retrieved the raw data from the MySQL database server, calculated the features and stored them again to the MySQL database server using a moving time window.

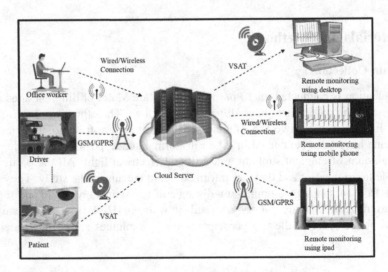

Fig. 1. Remote monitoring of HRV framework

A webpage is developed using PHP and Java script to present the features in real-time from remote places. A framework of remote monitoring is shown in Fig. 1.

2.2.1 Color Signal Pre-processing

Face detection is performed using Viola and Jones algorithm for each frame and region of interest (ROI) is selected from facial part where 80% of height and 60% of width of face is selected for ROI. Then KLT (Kanade-Lucas-Thomasi) algorithm is used to facial tracking for all consecutive frames. First RGB color values are extracted from ROI and the procedure is presented in Fig. 2. The RGB color values are converted into Lab color space. Lab color space has three independent color signals which are L, a and b where L represents the lightness of the images, a and b represents other color channels [2]. The advantage of Lab color space is that it is device independent and able to filter environmental illumination. To consider environmental illumination, another signal ab is constructed using only color signal a and b and signal L is discarded. This ab signal is able to filter ambient illumination.

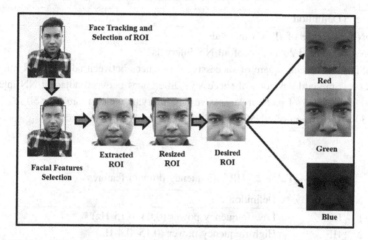

Fig. 2. Color signal extraction from facial images (Color figure online)

2.2.2 HR, IBI and HRV Feature Extraction

Human eyes cannot see the variation of facial color caused by cardiovascular system for each heart beat and hence a non-contact computer program is developed to detect color variation from where HR and IBI is calculated [1, 2, 18, 19].

Based on Lab color space the raw color signal ab is normalized and filtered using band pass filter [40–120 Hz]. Three algorithms such as FFT, ICA and PCA are used to extract HR and IBI from the lab color channel ab and then the average value is obtained. An example of major peaks and IBI are shown in Fig. 3. HRV features are calculated both in time domain and frequency domain. Definition of Time Domain Features and Frequency Domain Features are shown in Tables 1 and 2 respectively.

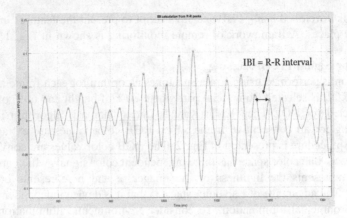

Fig. 3. Major peaks: IBI indicates time interval between two consecutive peaks

Table 1. HRV time domain features

No	Feature	Definition
1	meanNN	Average of all NN intervals
2	SDNN	Standard deviations of all NN intervals
3	RMSSD	Root mean square of successive differences between adjacent NN intervals
4	SDSD	Standard deviation of successive differences between adjacent NN intervals
5	NN50	Number of pairs of successive NN intervals which more than 50 ms
6	pNN50	Proportion of NN50 divided by total number of NN intervals

Table 2. HRV frequency domain features

No	Feature	Definition
1	LF	Low frequency power (0.04–0.15 Hz)
2	HF	High frequency power (0.15–0.4 Hz)
3	TotalPower	The variance of NN intervals over temporal segment
4	LF/HF ratio	Ratio of LF to HF

3   Results and Evaluation

The raw camera data is segmented into three parts each for one minute and HR is calculated from number of major peaks for each minute using FFT, ICA and PCA and then average HR of these three algorithms are taken. Therefore, for each subject we obtain three HR for minute one, two and three respectively. Then statistical parameters MAX, MIN, AVG, STD and MEDIAN of three HR of each subject are calculated. All these statistical parameters are also calculated for cStress measurement which are presented in Table 3 for ten subjects both for camera and sensor. For test subject 1, the statistical parameters of MAX, MIN, AVG, STD and MEDIAN of HR for sensor is 78,

Table 3. Statistical measurements of HR of three minute camera and cStress data

Test subject	MAX		MIN		AVG		STD		MEDIAN	
	Sensor	Camera	Sensor	Camera	Sensor	Camera	Sensor	Camera	Sensor	Camera
1	78	77	75	74	76.33	75.67	1.53	1.53	76	76
2	78	77	76	75	77.00	76.00	1.00	1.00	77	76
3	56	55	54	54	55.33	54.67	1.15	0.58	56	55
4	76	71	66	69	69.67	70.00	5.51	1.00	67	70
5	72	71	71	69	71.67	69.67	0.58	1.15	72	69
6	83	82	81	82	82.33	82.00	1.15	0.00	83	82
7	66	65	62	64	63.33	64.67	2.31	0.58	62	65
8	62	60	57	59	59.33	59.67	2.52	0.58	59	60
9	62	61	56	58	58.33	59.33	3.21	1.53	57	59
10	84	81	79	80	81.33	80.33	2.52	0.58	81	80
AVG (10 Subjects)	71.7	70	67.7	68.4	69.47	69.20	2.15	0.85	69	69.2

75, 76.33, 1.53 and 76 and for camera is 77, 74, 75.67, 1.53 and 76 which are closely related. The statistical parameters of other test subject also show that both sensor and camera parameters are closely related.

To calculate HRV features both in time domain and frequency domain first IBI is calculated for three minutes both for sensor and camera where sampling frequency of sensor and camera are 4 Hz and 12 Hz respectively. In time domain, statistical methods are applied on the Inter-beat-interval (IBI) signals to extract average of all NN intervals (meanNN), standard deviation of RR intervals (SDNN), root mean square of the all successive RR interval difference (RMSSD), standard deviation of differences between adjacent NN intervals (SDSD), number of pairs of adjacent NN intervals differing by more than 50 ms (NN50) features and percentage of NN50 count (pNN50). All these HRV time domain features are calculated and presented in Table 4.

Table 4. Comparison between sensor and camera system on time domain features.

Subject	meanNN		SDNN		RMSSD		SDSD		NN50		pNN50	
	Sensor	Camera	Sensor	Camera	Sensor	Camera	Sensor	Camera	Sensor	Camera	Sensor	Camera
1	785.81	799.15	35.35	36.44	7.12	12.34	7.11	12.35	0	0	0	0
2	778.22	791.17	24.51	25.43	8.16	12.79	8.16	12.80	2	2	0.36	0.35
3	1075.45	1088.53	34.17	34.94	7.83	13.00	7.83	13.00	1	1	0.13	0.12
4	864.05	877.11	74.41	74.84	15.08	18.22	15.08	18.22	10	12	1.60	1.90
5	833.72	846.66	37.69	38.47	9.14	13.69	9.13	13.69	0	1	0	0.16
6	727.03	740.19	35.01	35.39	9.68	14.01	9.68	14.01	0	3	0	0.56
7	941.78	954.90	39.06	39.79	9.31	13.87	9.31	13.87	2	4	0.29	0.58
8	1014.27	1027.23	68.89	69.01	23.09	25.59	23.09	25.59	38	47	5.20	6.35
9	1040.77	1053.99	133.61	134.00	55.04	55.89	55.04	55.89	97	91	12.94	11.99
10	735.75	749.17	41.54	41.89	14.01	17.52	14.01	17.52	10	11	1.88	2.03
AVG of 10 subjects	879.68	892.81	52.42	53.02	15.84	19.69	15.85	19.69	16	17.2	2.24	2.40

For frequency domain features, first IBI is transformed into frequency domain using FFT and PSD (power spectral density) is calculated considering 1024 FFT points. Then HRV frequency features such as Low frequency power (LF) (0.04–0.15 Hz), high frequency power (HF) (0.15–0.4 Hz), total power, and Ratio of LF to HF (LF/HF) are calculated and presented in Table 5. From Table 5 it is shown that frequency domain features both for sensor and camera are closely related.

Table 5. Comparison between sensor and camera system on frequency domain features.

Subject	LF		HF		TotalPower		LFHFratio	
	Sensor	Camera	Sensor	Camera	Sensor	Camera	Sensor	Camera
1	299.97	298.95	81.67	79.55	10264.78	10155.75	3.67	3.75
2	313.54	313.62	77.22	74.13	10055.41	9959.33	4.06	4.23
3	571.20	568.18	139.17	133.88	19210.03	18861.68	4.10	4.24
4	389.56	390.31	111.07	106.64	12471.12	12321.39	3.50	3.66
5	370.51	371.53	82.215	78.11	11555.06	11429.71	4.50	4.75
6	272.59	274.47	54.52	52.68	8787.64	8738.05	4.99	5.20
7	453.36	451.65	96.97	93.68	14747.83	14522.22	4.67	4.82
8	519.04	512.64	125.54	124.14	17118.14	16838.19	4.13	4.12
9	649.06	641.84	204.97	215.56	18125.50	17831.36	3.16	2.97
10	268.11	271.74	74.38	69.83	8997.96	8931.53	3.60	3.89
AVG of 10 subjects	410.69	409.49	104.77	102.82	13133.35	12958.92	4.04	4.16

4   Conclusion

The paper presented an approach for a non-contact based remote HRV monitoring using camera. Here, Lab color space approach is applied to extract physiological parameters from video recordings of the human face using a simple webcam with ambient daylight providing illumination. Both the time domain and frequency domain HRV features are extracted based on IBI and compared with a reference sensor system. Currently, the system is running in a local computer where HRV features are monitored via website in offline. However, the development of a real-time, remote, multi-physiological parameters measurement platform based on the proposed approach is ongoing.

Acknowledgement. The authors would like to acknowledge the Swedish Knowledge Foundation (KKS), Hök instrument AB, Volvo Car Corporation (VCC), The Swedish National Road and Transport Research Institute (VTI), Autoliv AB, Prevas AB Sweden, Hässlögymnasiets, Västerås and all the test subjects for their support of the research projects in this area.

References

1. Rahman, H., Ahmed, M.U., Begum, S.: Non-contact physiological parameters extraction using camera. In: The 1st Workshop on Embedded Sensor Systems for Health through Internet of Things (ESS-H IoT), October 2015
2. Rahman, H., Ahmed, M.U., Begum, S.: Non-contact heart rate monitoring using lab color space. In: 13th International Conference on Wearable, Micro & Nano Technologies for Personalized Health (pHealth2016), Crete, Greece, 29–31 May 2016
3. Qi, Z., Guo-qing, X., Ming, W., Yimin, Z., Wei, F.: Webcam based non-contact real-time monitoring for the physiological parameters of drivers. In: 2014 IEEE 4th Annual International Conference on Cyber Technology in Automation, Control, and Intelligent Systems (CYBER), pp. 648–652 (2014)
4. Abildstrom, S.Z., Jensen, B.T., Agner, E., Torp-Pedersen, C., Nyvad, O.L.E., Wachtell, K., et al.: Heart rate versus heart rate variability in risk prediction after myocardial infarction. J. Cardiovasc. Electrophysiol. **14**, 168–173 (2003)
5. Kleiger, R.E., Miller, J.P., Bigger Jr., J.T., Moss, A.J.: Decreased heart rate variability and its association with increased mortality after acute myocardial infarction. Am. J. Cardiol. **59**, 256–262 (1987)
6. Tsunoda, K., Chiba, A., Chigira, H., Yoshida, K., Watanabe, T., Mizuno, O.: Online estimation of a cognitive performance using heart rate variability. In: 2016 38th Annual International Conference of the IEEE Engineering in Medicine and Biology Society (EMBC), pp. 761–765 (2016)
7. McDuff, D., Gontarek, S., Picard, R.: Remote measurement of cognitive stress via heart rate variability. In: 2014 36th Annual International Conference of the IEEE Engineering in Medicine and Biology Society, pp. 2957–2960 (2014)
8. Bousefsaf, F., Maaoui, C., Pruski, A.: Remote assessment of the heart rate variability to detect mental stress. In: 2013 7th International Conference on Pervasive Computing Technologies for Healthcare (PervasiveHealth), pp. 348–351 (2013)
9. Bousefsaf, F., Maaoui, C., Pruski, A.: Remote assessment of physiological parameters by non-contact technologies to quantify and detect mental stress states. In: 2014 International Conference on Control, Decision and Information Technologies (CoDIT), pp. 719–723 (2014)
10. Kranjec, J., Beguš, S., Geršak, G., Drnovšek, J.: Non-contact heart rate and heart rate variability measurements: a review. Biomed. Sig. Process. Control **13**, 102–112 (2014)
11. Parnandi, A., Gutierrez-Osuna, R.: Contactless measurement of heart rate variability from pupillary fluctuations. In: 2013 Humaine Association Conference on Affective Computing and Intelligent Interaction (ACII), pp. 191–196 (2013)
12. Peng, R.C., Zhou, X.L., Lin, W.H., Zhang, Y.T.: Extraction of heart rate variability from smartphone photoplethysmograms. Comput. Math. Methods Med. **2015**, 1–11 (2015)
13. Tasli, H.E., Gudi, A., den Uyl, M.: Remote PPG based vital sign measurement using adaptive facial regions. In: 2014 IEEE International Conference on Image Processing (ICIP), pp. 1410–1414 (2014)
14. Parnandi, A., Gutierrez-Osuna, R.: Contactless measurement of heart rate variability from pupillary fluctuations. In: 2013 Humaine Association Conference on Affective Computing and Intelligent Interaction, pp. 191–196 (2013)
15. Li, X., Chen, J., Zhao, G., Pietikainen, M.: Remote heart rate measurement from face videos under realistic situations. In: 2014 IEEE Conference on Computer Vision and Pattern Recognition (CVPR), pp. 4264–4271 (2014)

16. Verkruysse, W., Svaasand, L.O., Nelson, J.S.: Remote plethysmographic imaging using ambient light. Opt. Express **16**, 21434–21445 (2008)
17. Zhao, F., Li, M., Qian, Y., Tsien, J.Z.: Remote measurements of heart and respiration rates for telemedicine. PLoS ONE **8**, e71384 (2013)
18. Rahman, H., Begum, S., Ahmed, M.U., Funk, P.: Real time heart rate monitoring from facial RGB color video using webcam. In: 29th Annual Workshop of the Swedish Artificial Intelligence Society (SAIS), Malmö, Sweden (2016)
19. Rahman, H., Iyer, S., Meusburger, C., Dobrovoljski, K., Stoycheva, M., Turkulov, V., et al.: SmartMirror: an embedded non-contact system for health monitoring at home. Presented at the the 3rd EAI International Conference on IoT Technologies for HealthCare (Healthy-IoT-2016), Västerås, Sweden, 18–19 October 2016
20. Ahmed, M.U.: An intelligent healthcare service to monitor vital signs in daily life – a case study on health-IoT. Int. J. Eng. Res. Appl. (IJERA) **7**(3), 43–55 (2017)
21. Ahmed, M.U., Björkman, M., Causevic, A., Fotouhi, H., Lindén, M.: An overview on the internet of things for health monitoring systems. In: 2nd EAI International Conference on IoT Technologies for HealthCare (HealthyIoT2015), October 2015
22. Ahmed, M.U.: A personalized health-monitoring system for elderly by combining rules and case-based reasoning. In: 12th International Conference on Wearable Micro and Nano Technologies for Personalized Health (pHealth 2015), June 2015
23. Ahmed, M.U., Espinosa, J.R., Reissner, A., Domingo, À., Banaee, H., Loutfi, A., Rafael-Palou, X.: Self-serve ICT-based health monitoring to support active ageing. In: 8th International Conference on Health Informatics (HEALTHINF), January 2015

How Accurate Are Smartphone Accelerometers to Identify Intermittent Claudication?

Carole Frindel[(✉)] and David Rousseau

Univ. Lyon, INSA-Lyon, Université Claude Bernard Lyon 1, CNRS, Inserm,
CREATIS UMR 5220, U1206, 69621 Lyon, France
`carole.frindel@creatis.insa-lyon.fr`

Abstract. Claudication is a cramping pain that is worsened by walking and relieved with rest. It is caused by inadequate blood flow to the leg muscles because of atherosclerosis. Recently, smartphones and their sensors have been proposed in the context of mobile health to monitor gait. However, their use remains disputed: objections concern the quality of the collected data. Therefore, the work presented in this paper proposes to study three main sources of noise observed in smartphone accelerometers and to objectively assess their impact on claudication detection. To do so, we first observe three noise sources in four different smartphones to get an idea of their ranges; we second compare the smartphones' signals to a ground truth from a vision-based system and third propose to detect claudication by estimating duty cycle from the vertical accelerometer signal and to evaluate the impact of the three noise sources on this basis.

Keywords: Intermittent claudication · Smartphone · Accelerometer
Human motion · Gait analysis · Motion tracking

1 Introduction

Injury to a lower limb may disrupt natural walking. In intermittent claudication, significant differences can be observed in kinematic parameters as cadence, stance and swing times and step width when compared with healthy controls [1,2]. Hence, an accurate motion tracking system is needed to observe these differences. Several human motion tracking systems exist. The most famous are vision-based systems made popular from applications in sport analysis [3,4] and lead to the 3D localization of the patient's limbs by combining the data of several cameras. Markerless systems [5] follow the patient's contours while marker-based systems, such as VICON [6], follow either light-reflecting markers or light-emitting diodes attached to the patient. Such systems enable precise localization but they are expensive, cumbersome and therefore can not be used in outpatient care units or at home. Recently, smartphones and their sensors have been proposed to address theses problems [7]. In smartphone-based systems, the

© ICST Institute for Computer Sciences, Social Informatics and Telecommunications Engineering 2018
M. U. Ahmed et al. (Eds.): HealthyIoT 2017, LNICST 225, pp. 19–25, 2018.
https://doi.org/10.1007/978-3-319-76213-5_3

patient carries a smartphone and uses its sensors to capture his motion without interfering with his natural behavior [8,9] by integrating measurements of a GPS, accelerometer and/or gyroscope. Nevertheless, the use of smartphones and their low-cost sensors remains controversial in the medical community. Although the miniaturized and non-invasive aspect is attractive, objections concern the quality of the collected data as well as the reliability of the associated software technologies in a clinical context. In this context, our work addresses three issues. The first one aims to characterize three main sources of noise (sampling jitter, rate and quantification) observed in the accelerometers of smartphones to assess their ranges. The second one seeks to build a ground truth from a high frame rate video camera for comparison with the signals from the smartphones. Finally, the third one evaluates from the degraded signals (according to the characteristics identified in the first section) of the ground truth (built in the second section) the detection capacities for claudication.

2   Noise Study

Concerning the noise, we decided to study three characteristics: the quantification for which the information is readily available on the web, the sampling rate and jitter that can be easily obtained from simple acquisitions. Other sources of electronic noise (thermal noise, shot noise, flicker noise) have not been considered because they are much more difficult to estimate. In order to study the noise characteristics of the smartphone accelerometers, we had four different devices at our disposal: respectively a Samsung S6 (380 euros), a Samsung A5 (270 euros), a Samsung A3 (220 euros) and a LG Optimus F6 (130 euros).

Quantification. Most of the sensors in smartphones are MEMS (Microelectromechanical systems) based. The ADXL335 and ADXL345 are two of the most popular. According to their technical documentation [10], the output precision varies from 8 bits to 13 bits.

Sampling Rate. To estimate the sampling rate we performed experiments on the different devices. To do so, an Android program has been developed to consult, for each measurement, the system clock of the smartphone accelerometer and therefore to calculate a posteriori the delay between each measurement. On average, the sampling rates recorded for the different devices are respectively 15 Hz for the Samsung A5 and A3, 20 Hz for the LG Optimus F6 and adaptative sampling rate (maximum limit 50 Hz) for the Samsung S6.

Sampling Jitter. To estimate the sampling jitter we relied on the same experiments that for the sampling rate. For each device, time evolution, distribution and autocorrelation of the centered sampling jitter is illustrated in Fig. 1. The different devices behave differently regarding the sampling jitter. Galaxy A5, Galaxy A3 and LG Optimus F6 present a sampling jitter which is very closed to

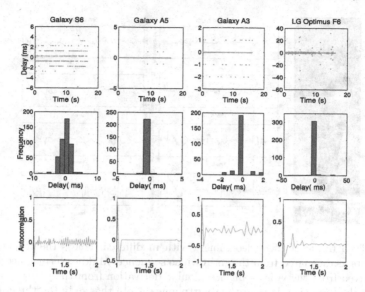

Fig. 1. Each column is for a different device. First line: time evolution; second line: distribution; third line: autocorrelation of the sampling jitter. Data were previously centered.

a Dirac distribution, where Samsung S6 presents the largest dispersion around the Dirac. The jitter of these three devices can be modeled by a white noise in accordance with their autocorrelation. Surprisingly, the Samsung S6 which has an adaptive sampling rate does not have the same shape of distribution for the jitter: its distribution is more like a generalized Gaussian and its autocorrelation indicates a deterministic and cyclic jitter which may come from a timer in the adaptation process.

3   Ground Truth from Vision-Based System

Subjects. Four healthy volunteers without any known gait pathology participated in the walking experiments. During the tests, they were asked to walk on a treadmill for 2 min: the first minute at 1.2 km/h and the second minute at 2.4 km/h. Then the subject realized exactly the same session with a knee splint.

Reference System. Validation of the accelerometer signals and extracted features was performed against a high frame rate video camera (Gige Vision). The motion tracking is based on markers that were placed on the different segments of the leg (respectively hip, thigh, ankle and foot) as illustrated on Fig. 2. On these same segments, the four different devices presented in Sect. 2 have been

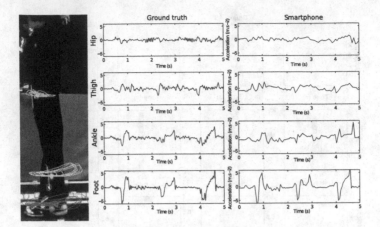

Fig. 2. Left: a frame of the video camera with in different colors the trajectories of the segments as estimated from the entire video sequence. Middle: vertical acceleration signals derived from the video sequence (double derivation from the positions). Right: vertical acceleration signals from the smartphones. Note that only the three first gait cycles of the 2 min test are displayed.

fastened (hip = Samsung A3; thigh = Samsung A5; ankle = LG Optimus; foot = Samsung S6). The video camera was placed close to the treadmill such that the pointing direction is approximately perpendicular to the sagittal plan to avoid distorsions. During each gait test, we collected simultaneous video at 300 Hz and acceleration signals in 3D at sampling rate indicated in Sect. 2 for hip, thigh, ankle and foot. The motion tracking from the video sequence was performed using an open-source tracking software [11]. Markers that were placed an the leg segments were automatically detected using local features detector (Laplacian of Gaussian): it requires to calibrate in size the frames of the video sequence and give an estimate of the size of the markers to be searched.

4   Claudication Detection

A number of spatio-temporal parameters of gait have been proposed over the years to detect claudication [1,2]: step length, step duration, stance phase, load response, single support, pre-swing, and swing phase (%). In this work, we propose to resume these in one indicator: the duty cycle (DC) of the periodic walking function. As illustrated on Fig. 3, the acceleration signal has to be binarized: from the vertical acceleration signal, the algorithm detects time intervals during which accelerometer is at rest (0) and vice versa (1). More precisely, the binarization was based on z-score: if a new acceleration is below a fixed signed number of standard deviations (3 in our case) from the mean (estimated over three gait cycles) then it is considered as at rest. DC is expressed as the ratio of the duration of the swing phase (1) over the total duration of the step.

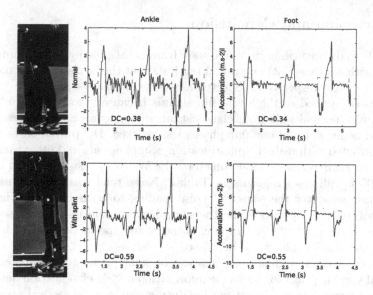

Fig. 3. First row: normal walk. Second row: walk with knee splint. Middle column: ground truth acceleration signals from the ankle segment. Right column: ground truth acceleration signals from the foot segment. Averaged DC for the 2 min test is given for each condition in the lower left angle of the graph. Note that only the three first gait cycles are displayed.

Table 1. Averaged DC and standard deviation computed for the 2 min test regarding the different sources of noise for the foot. For each line, the other sources of noise are fixed: quantification, sampling rate and jitter studies are carried out with respectively 50 Hz and no jitter, 13 bits and no jitter and 13 bits and 50 Hz.

# Bits	13	12	11	10	9	8
Normal	0.338 ± 0.002	0.338 ± 0.002	0.338 ± 0.002	0.337 ± 0.003	0.328 ± 0.005	0.321 ± 0.011
With splint	0.523 ± 0.002	0.523 ± 0.002	0.523 ± 0.003	0.521 ± 0.003	0.510 ± 0.012	0.505 ± 0.023
Rate	50	40	30	20	10	
Normal	0.338 ± 0.002	0.328 ± 0.005	0.327 ± 0.015	0.315 ± 0.022	0.303 ± 0.030	
With splint	0.523 ± 0.002	0.519 ± 0.009	0.517 ± 0.025	0.506 ± 0.031	0.483 ± 0.039	
Jitter	S6	A5	A3	F6		
Normal	0.3204 ± 0.021	0.3294 ± 0.004	0.3305 ± 0.003	0.3232 ± 0.023		
With splint	0.5010 ± 0.033	0.5150 ± 0.064	0.5152 ± 0.071	0.5061 ± 0.037		

In order to measure the impact of the three noise sources on DC, we simulated degraded signals from the ground-truth accelerometer signals for observed ranges in Sect. 2. In other words, ground truth signals were sampled by the appropriate factor, quantified on the adequate number of bits and jittered by the four distributions given in Fig. 1 to aim the observed ranges. The analysis of DC regarding the different noise sources (see Table 1) has to be done in comparison with DC observed in ground truth (see Fig. 3).

5   Discussion and Conclusion

DC is able to distinguish normal free walk from constrained walk (miming claudication with a knee splint) on ground truth data at the levels of ankle and foot: the Welch's t-test respectively reported a p-value of 1.18e−4 and 3.16e−05. DC has not been applied to thigh and hip signals because it was not significative to distinguish normal walk from claudication: these signals have smaller amplitudes and hence flat and non-flat phases less marked. DC proved to be robust when confronted with realistic quantification, sampling rate and jitter variability observed on smartphones's accelerometers: the Welch's t-test reported a p-value below 0.05 for all cases reported in Table 1. Noise tend to under evaluate the swing phase whatever the source of noise leading to a smaller DC. The most critical noise source appears to be the sampling rate and its impacts seems to be greater with splint: if the sampling is too coarse, peaks of acceleration constituting the non-flat phase can be missed.

We presented an original noise analysis of smartphone accelerometers from devices of varying prices for a specific informational task: claudication detection. Claudication was detected by estimating duty cycle from the vertical accelerometer signal. Three noise sources were investigated: sampling jitter, sampling rate and quantification. Validation of this study was based on ground-truth from high frame rate video camera. Our results demonstrate for the first time that smartphones' sensors are sufficiently accurate to detect claudication. This pilot study opens interesting perspectives: state-of-the-art methods for claudication detection could be compared to determine which one is the most robust to the typical noises identified in this study; and smartphones' sensors could be tested to detect other walking irregularities.

References

1. Chen, S.J., Pipinos, I., Johanning, J., Radovic, M., Huisinga, J.M., Myers, S.A., Stergiou, N.: Bilateral claudication results in alterations in the gait biomechanics at the hip and ankle joints. J. Biomech. **41**, 2506–2514 (2008)
2. Koutakis, P., Johanning, J.M., Haynatzki, G.R., Myers, S.A., Stergiou, N., Longo, G.M., Pipinos, I.I.: Abnormal joint powers before and after the onset of claudication symptoms. J. Vasc. Surg. **52**, 340–347 (2010)
3. Barris, S., Button, C.: A review of vision-based motion analysis in sport. Sports Med. **38**, 1025–1043 (2008)
4. Thomas, G., Gade, R., Moeslund, T.B., Carr, P., Hilton, A.: Computer vision for sports: current applications and research topics. Comput. Vis. Image Underst. **159**, 3–18 (2017)
5. Gonzlez-Ortega, D., Daz-Pernas, F.J., Martnez-Zarzuela, M., Antn-Rodrguez, M., Dez-Higuera, J.F., Boto-Giralda, D.: Real-time hands, face and facial features detection and tracking: application to cognitive rehabilitation tests monitoring. J. Netw. Comput. Appl. **33**, 447–466 (2010)
6. VICON, May 2017. http://www.vicon.com
7. Khambati, H.K., Boles, K., Jetty, P.: Google maps offers a new way to evaluate claudication. J. Vasc. Surg. **65**, 1467–1472 (2017)

8. Yang, C.-C., Hsu, Y.-L.: A review of accelerometry-based wearable motion detectors for physical activity monitoring. Sensors **10**, 7772–7788 (2010)
9. Patel, S., Park, H., Bonato, P., Chan, L., Rodgers, M.: A review of wearable sensors and systems with application in rehabilitation. J. Neuroeng. Rehabil. **9**, 1–17 (2012)
10. ADX345, May 2017. http://www.analog.com/media/en/technical-documentation/data-sheets/ADXL345.pdf
11. TrackMate, May 2017. http://imagej.net/TrackMate

Distributed Multivariate Physiological Signal Analytics for Drivers' Mental State Monitoring

Shaibal Barua[(⊠)](ID), Mobyen Uddin Ahmed(ID),
and Shahina Begum(ID)

School of Innovation, Design and Engineering,
Mälardalen University, 72123 Västerås, Sweden
shaibal.barua@mdh.se

Abstract. This paper presents a distributed data analytics approach for drivers' mental state monitoring using multivariate physiological signals. Driver's mental states such as cognitive distraction, sleepiness, stress, etc. can be fatal contributing factors and to prevent car crashes these factors need to be understood. Here, a cloud-based approach with heterogeneous sensor sources that generates extremely large data sets of physiological signals need to be handled and analysed in a big data scenario. In the proposed physiological big data analytics approach, for driver state monitoring, heterogeneous data coming from multiple sources i.e., multivariate physiological signals are used, processed and analyzed to aware impaired vehicle drivers. Here, in a distributed big data environment, multi-agent case-based reasoning facilitates parallel case similarity matching and handles data that are coming from single and multiple physiological signal sources.

Keywords: Physiological signals · Distributed analytics
Case-based reasoning

1 Introduction

While driving, cognitive distractions occur when a driver keeps his/her eye on the road and hands on the steering, yet takes the mind off from the driving task, such as hands-free cell phone calls, listening to the radio, and even having a conversation with fellow passenger. The concern of driving performance contemplating cognitively loading activities on traffic safety is addressed in [1, 2, 20]. Driving is a proactive task that requires anticipation and adaptation with respect to the road users' behaviours, and their actions are revolving all the time. This whole process of driving can be seen as a nearly automated, partially self-paced and satisficing task [3] and to anticipate safe travel plan and goal full attention is required from the driver. Hence, for the futuristic automated transportation and new theory of driver distraction it is important to determine the cognitive driving distraction and the contribution factors of inattention while driving, which can prevent happening bad things.

Physiological signals became reliable and most useful over the years in identifying driver's cognitive distraction. The advancement of wearable sensor technology makes it possible to collect tremendous amount of data with various variation which also

© ICST Institute for Computer Sciences, Social Informatics and Telecommunications Engineering 2018
M. U. Ahmed et al. (Eds.): HealthyIoT 2017, LNICST 225, pp. 26–33, 2018.
https://doi.org/10.1007/978-3-319-76213-5_4

becomes the part of big data biological process and it requires trade-off between resources, to handle the stream of sensor data [4]. Issues that arise in the big data biological process such as data are frequently reside in distributed data platforms, often data are too large to fit in a single memory, and single thread processing is not sufficient to regulate the growing computational volume and complexity [5, 6]. The big data biological process can be leveraged through distributed analytics using machine learning. However, currently there are few distributed platforms available for predictive analytics and most machine learning are not embarrassingly parallel. For example, case-based reasoning (CBR) is a reasoner that solves a new problem by remembering and using previously solved problems that are similar to the current problem, thus avoids the re-invent the wheel approach. However, CBR examines individual cases in a sequence to find the most similar cases, which constrains parallelization. In big data paradigm, multi-agent CBR architecture can be beneficial for organizing knowledge base within the system and processing knowledge by the system [7, 18, 19].

This paper presents a distributed analytics approach for drivers' mental state monitoring in terms of cognitive distraction using multivariate physiological signals. Physiological sensors signal used in the analytics are Electrooculogram (EOG), Pupil Diameter, Electroencephalogram (EEG), Electrogastrogram (EGG), respiration, and Skin Conductance. In the study, the Attention Selection Model (ASM) [8] is considered to detect the effect of cognitive distraction on traffic safety. The ASM is a conceptual model of attention selection and multitasking in everyday natural driving situations, where attention selection is acknowledged as a form of adaptive behavior, rather than consequence of limited capacity. Reflecting the ASM model a version of n-back task [9] is adapted as a cognitively loading secondary task.

2 Materials and Methods

The vehicle driver monitoring study was performed in an advanced moving-base simulator (SIM III[1]) at VTI in Linköping. This moving based simulator has the ability to simulate movements and forces that act upon natural driving by allowing motion in four degrees of freedom, and the platform can simulate vibrations and smaller movements. Data acquisition was performed using DeweSoft S-box 2[2] computer with analog terminals and in the simulation control computer. The physiological signals were recorded using g.tec system, where g.tec plugin was connected to the S-box. Physiological signals were recorded from 36 male participants with no known disease and medication; aged between 35 to 50 years and having driving license for more than 10 years. The scenarios in the simulator were design as rural road with one lane in each direction, some curves and slopes, and a speed limit of 80 km/h. For this cognitive distraction study, driving environment in the simulator was consisted of three reoccurring scenarios: four way crossing, a hidden exit on the right side of the road with a warning sign, and a strong side wind in open terrain [10]. A secondary task (auditory 1-back task) was deployed in two occasions in each scenario.

---

[1] https://www.vti.se/en/research-areas/vtis-driving-simulators/.

[2] www.dewesoft.com.

The sample size of the physiological signals was 256 Hz and six different physiological signals were recorded. Besides, 30 channels EEG system was used in the data collection. All these produce a large amount of data in long run and each of the signal has different characteristics for example, rapid changes of EEG, where ECG and skin conductance signals have slow fluctuation. Thus, the sample set requires consideration of 3 V's of big data: *Volume*, *Variety* and *Veracity*. Moreover, the data value from different signals often needs to handle differently. Again, considering real-time monitoring of cognitive distraction the *Velocity* of the data needs to be handled.

2.1 Distributed Analytics Approach

To handle and analyse such big data set for vehicle driver monitoring a cloud-based distributed analytics approach is proposed. A schematic diagram of the big data (i.e. distributed multivariate physiological signal) analytics for drivers' state monitoring is shown in Fig. 1. The approach is comprised of several cloud modules/nodes namely data storage, data processing and analytics platform. All forms of recorded data are transferred from the local computer to the data storage via Internet.

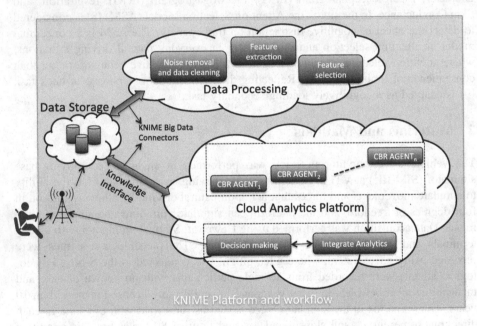

Fig. 1. Schematic diagram of the proposed distributed analytics system

The KNIME Platform and server[3] are used to develop the workflow and its big data extensions are used to connect the data storage and analytics platform. CBR agents, noise handling, feature extraction, and feature selections are done in Matlab scripting

---

[3] https://www.knime.com/.

and KNIME's community nodes were used to integrate them in the KNIME workflow. KNIME Big Data Connectors and KNIME Cluster Executor are two node libraries that enable to work within Hadoop ecosystem such as Hive and Impala. Data storage i.e., import and export of data and SQL are handled using the KNIME Big Data Connectors. The data distribution and analytics are distributed among the KNIME clusters through KNIME Cluster Executor, which provides a slim connection layer between KNIME Analytics Platform and computing cluster.

One of the important tasks in any data analytics is to ensure the quality of the data. Here, a cloud-based data processing module is considered, which mainly performs the noise handling and data cleaning. Since each physiological signal affects differently, it requires different algorithms for different analytics. In this study, for the EEG signals a fully automated EEG artifacts handling algorithm [11] has been developed. Other methods such as moving average filtering is used to remove noise from skin conductance and pupil diameter signals, EOG signal is filtered with a median filters, ECG can be cleaned using [12], etc. Another key component for analytics is the representations of data for specific problem domain. It requires a feature extraction and selection of sub-modules. Features are extracted from all kinds of signals, and stored for the data analytics. Table 1 represents the list of features extracted from the physiological signals.

The cloud analytics platform is comprised of multi-agent case-based reasoning (CBR). CBR system comprises of sub-tasks such as case base maintenance, cases retrieval, cases adaptation and retaining new cases [13], where distributed CBR can achieve maximum efficiency for big data. In distributed CBR research, multiple agent CBR systems are widely used and well establish for managing the CBR sub-tasks [14, 21].

Table 1. Features extracted from physiological signals.

Signals	Extracted features
EEG	**Frequency:** Power Spectral Density (PSD) of delta (0–4 Hz), theta (4–8 Hz), alpha (8–13 Hz), beta (13–30 Hz), and gamma (30–50 Hz) [10] **Time:** Hurst Exponent, three Hjorth descriptors, kurtosis, auto mutual information, sample entropy, permutation entropy, and approximate entropy [10]
EOG	Number of blinks, blink time, standard deviation of amplitude [15]
Respiration	Respiration rate
Pupil diameter	Average pupil diameter [16]
Skin conductance	**Frequency:** average power of the signal under 1 Hz [16] **Time:** mean value, standard deviation, mean of normalised signal, standard deviation of normalised signal, means of absolute values of the first and second differences in normalised signal, sum of Peak magnitudes, peak duration, number of peaks, time to peak [16]
ECG	**Frequency:** Power spectral destiny of very low (≤ 0.04 Hz), low (0.04–0.15 Hz), high (0.15–0.4 Hz) and ratio low and high frequency power [17] **Time:** mean and standard deviation RR peak, mean heart rate, SDNN, RMSSD, NN50 Count, and pNN50 [17] **Nonlinear:** Dispersion of the points perpendicular and along to the axis of line of identity Alpha of total slop, short and long-range scaling exponent

In the proposed approach, each CBR agent can be called to perform the classification task either for individual signals or a combination of signals. This depends on how the case library is requested from the data storage. Thus, it reduces the feature vector size of the cases. Moreover, when a new case arrives distributed case libraries can append only that new case to them, which supports the parallel classification. Hence, knowledge bases are distributed across several nodes in clusters using the multiple agents. Then the only overhead is to integrate the results from the multiple agents using *Integrate Analytics* sub module. This provides the freedom to choose type of analytics i.e., using individualized knowledge or combination of knowledge for decision-making. Consequently, this approach tackles the sub-tasks require by CBR and other needs of the big data processing such as noise handling, anomaly detection condition monitoring etc.

3   Results

Case libraries reside in the data storage. Here the cases are labeled based on the 1-back task was performed or not. Each multi-agent CBR retrieves most similar cases that have similarity $\geq 90\%$, using a Euclidian distance-based similarity matching function. The *Integrate Analytics* sub module collects all the similar cases and then applies a majority voting to choose the most similar case. For the evaluation of the CBR classification a leave-one-out approach is used for selecting the query cases. The evaluation was performed considering individual scenario and combination of different scenarios and the results are presented in Table 2.

Table 2. Summary of CBR classification considering individual scenario and combined scenario. Here, HE = Hidden exit scenario, CR = Crossing scenario, SW = side wind scenario, and All = case library containing cases from all scenarios.

Scenarios	Criteria							
	Total cases	True positive (TP)	False positive (FP)	False negative (FN)	True negative (TN)	Sensitivity = TP/ (TP + FN)	Specificity = TN/ (FP + TN)	Accuracy = (TP + TN)/ (P + N)
	EEG signals							
All	396	146	52	64	134	≈ 0.70	≈ 0.72	≈ 0.71
HE + CR	264	104	28	43	89	≈ 0.71	≈ 0.76	≈ 0.73
CR	132	49	17	19	47	≈ 0.72	≈ 0.73	≈ 0.73
HE	132	51	15	30	36	≈ 0.63	≈ 0.71	≈ 0.66
SW	132	53	13	19	47	≈ 0.71	≈ 0.78	≈ 0.76
	Combined other signals							
All	396	141	57	62	136	≈ 0.69	≈ 0.70	≈ 0.70
HE + CR	264	86	46	43	89	≈ 0.66	≈ 0.67	≈ 0.66
CR	132	49	17	26	40	≈ 0.65	≈ 0.70	≈ 0.67
HE	132	41	25	22	44	≈ 0.65	≈ 0.64	≈ 0.64
SW	132	47	19	16	50	≈ 0.75	≈ 0.72	≈ 0.75

It can be observed from Table 2 that for CBR classification, two case libraries were built one using the EEG signals and other using the combination of signals. The results show that for both EEG signals and combination of signals side wind scenario achieved better classification accuracy that is 76% and 75% respectively. Compare to the other signals, EEG signals based classification shows better performance, which suggests cognitive distraction may influence EEG signals better than other signals. The overall classification results is less than 80% and the reason might be that the 1-back task is easy for these drivers to perform and thus the differences are not sufficient enough to classify the load and normal states. However, it shows a preliminary investigation result using multi-agent CBR, which illustrates that distributed CBR classification has a good potential in big data context. However, further development is ongoing in terms of feature selection and decision fusion in the *Integrate Analytics* module to improve the classification results.

4 Summary

Cognitive distraction while driving is an important research area of traffic safety. Today, because of the wearable sensors availability, cloud computing, and IoT, datasets become huge in volume, with high velocity and also consist of large variety in characteristics. In this paper, we have considered a distributed data analytics approach to classify cognitive distraction using multivariate physiological signals in the cloud. Here, not only the data but also the analytical services are distributed in several modules in the cloud. The main CBR classification scheme is developed considering multi-agent technology. Multi-agent based distributed CBR has been long using, and in big data paradigm it can leverage over the increasing data volume and competence and contextualisation. The proposed multi-agent CBR approach can achieve parallelism in terms of running the same or different similarity function in parallel for large distributed case libraries. In this work only multi-agent based case retrieval is proposed, yet it opens several future directions such as the distributed adaptation for CBR, interface between case libraries and agents for distributed data.

Acknowledgments. The authors would like to acknowledge VINNOVA (Swedish Governmental Agency for Innovation Systems) for supporting the "Vehicle Driver Monitoring" project. The authors would also like to acknowledge our project partners Volvo Car Corporation and the Swedish National Road and Transport Research Institute (VTI).

References

1. Lee, J.D., Boyle, L.N.: Is talking to your car dangerous? It depends. Hum. Factors **57**(8), 1297–1299 (2015). https://doi.org/10.1177/0018720815610945
2. Caird, J.K., Willness, C.R., Steel, P., Scialfa, C.: A meta-analysis of the effects of cell phones on driver performance. Accid. Anal. Prev. **40**(4), 1282–1293 (2008). https://doi.org/10.1016/j.aap.2008.01.009
3. Kircher, K., Ahlstrom, C.: Minimum required attention. Hum. Factors 0018720816672756 (2016). https://doi.org/10.1177/0018720816672756

4. Baccarelli, E., Cordeschi, N., Mei, A., Panella, M., Shojafar, M., Stefa, J.: Energy-efficient dynamic traffic offloading and reconfiguration of networked data centers for big data stream mobile computing: review, challenges, and a case study. IEEE Netw. **30**(2), 54–61 (2016). https://doi.org/10.1109/MNET.2016.7437025

5. Leary, D.E.O.: Artificial intelligence and big data. IEEE Intell. Syst. **28**(2), 96–99 (2013). https://doi.org/10.1109/MIS.2013.39

6. Cuzzocrea, A., Song, I.-Y., Davis, K.C.: Analytics over large-scale multidimensional data: the big data revolution! Paper Presented at the Proceedings of the ACM 14th International Workshop on Data Warehousing and OLAP, Glasgow, Scotland, UK (2011)

7. Plaza, E., McGinty, L.: Distributed case-based reasoning. Knowl. Eng. Rev. **20**(3), 261–265 (2006). https://doi.org/10.1017/S0269888906000683

8. Engström, J., Victor, T., Markkula, G.: Attention selection and multitasking in everyday driving: a conceptual model (2013)

9. Kane, M.J., Conway, A.R.A., Miura, T.K., Colflesh, G.J.H.: Working memory, attention control, and the n-back task: a question of construct validity. J. Exp. Psychol. Learn. Mem. Cogn. **33**(3), 615–622 (2007)

10. Barua, S., Ahmed, M.U., Begum, S.: Classifying drivers' cognitive load using EEG signals. Stud. Health Technol. Inform. **237**, 99–106 (2017)

11. Barua, S., Begum, S., Ahmed, M.U.: Intelligent automated EEG artifacts handling using wavelet transform, independent component analysis and hierarchal clustering. In: Perego, P., Andreoni, G., Rizzo, G. (eds.) MobiHealth 2016. LNICST, vol. 192, pp. 144–148. Springer, Cham (2017). https://doi.org/10.1007/978-3-319-58877-3_19

12. Kaufmann, T., Sütterlin, S., Schulz, S.M., Vögele, C.: ARTiiFACT: a tool for heart rate artifact processing and heart rate variability analysis. Behav. Res. Methods **43**(4), 1161–1170 (2011). https://doi.org/10.3758/s13428-011-0107-7

13. Aamodt, A., Plaza, E.: Case-based reasoning: foundational issues, methodological variations, and system approaches. AI Commun. **7**(1), 39–59 (1994)

14. Reichle, M., Bach, K., Althoff, K.-D.: Knowledge engineering within the application-independent architecture SEASALT. Int. J. Knowl. Eng. Data Min. **1**(3), 202–215 (2011). https://doi.org/10.1504/ijkedm.2011.037643

15. Benedetto, S., Pedrotti, M., Minin, L., Baccino, T., Re, A., Montanari, R.: Driver workload and eye blink duration. Transp. Res. Part F Traffic Psychol. Behav. **14**(3), 199–208 (2011). https://doi.org/10.1016/j.trf.2010.12.001

16. Zhai, J., Barreto, A.: Stress detection in computer users based on digital signal processing of noninvasive physiological variables. In: 2006 International Conference of the IEEE Engineering in Medicine and Biology Society, 30 August 2006–3 September 2006, pp. 1355–1358 (2006)

17. Mehler, B., Reimer, B., Wang, Y.: A comparison of heart rate and heart rate variability indices in distinguishing single-task driving and driving under secondary cognitive workload. Paper Presented at the 6th International Driving Symposium on Human Factors in Driver Assessment, Training, and Vehicle Design, Olympic Valley - Lake Tahoe, California, USA, 27–30 June 2011

18. Begum, S., Barua, S., Filla, R., Ahmed, M.U.: Classification of physiological signals for wheel loader operators using multi-scale entropy analysis and case-based reasoning. Expert Syst. Appl. **41**(2), 295–305 (2014)

19. Ahmed, M.U., Begum, S., Funk, P.: A hybrid case-based system in stress diagnosis and treatment. In: IEEE-EMBS International Conference on Biomedical and Health Informatics (BHI2012) (2012)

20. Begum, S., Ahmed, M.U., Funk, P., Filla, R.: Mental state monitoring system for the professional drivers based on heart rate variability analysis. In: Computer Science and Information Systems (FedCSIS), pp. 35–42 (2012)
21. Begum, S., Barua, S., Ahmed, M.U.: Physiological sensor signals classification for healthcare using sensor data fusion and case-based reasoning. Sensors **14**(7), 11770–11785 (2014)

An Efficient Design of a Machine Learning-Based Elderly Fall Detector

L. P. Nguyen[1,2], M. Saleh[1,2], and R. Le Bouquin Jeannès[1,2(✉)]

[1] INSERM U1099, 35000 Rennes, France
regine.le-bouquin-jeannes@univ-rennes1.fr
[2] Université de Rennes 1, LTSI, 35000 Rennes, France

Abstract. Elderly fall detection is an important health care application as falls represent the major reason of injuries. An efficient design of a machine learning-based wearable fall detection system is proposed in this paper. The proposed system depends only on a 3-axial accelerometer to capture the elderly motion. As the power consumption is proportional to the sampling frequency, the performance of the proposed fall detector is analyzed as a function of this frequency in order to determine the best trade-off between performance and power consumption. Thanks to efficient extracted features, the proposed system achieves a sensitivity of 99.73% and a specificity of 97.7% using a 40 Hz sampling frequency notably outperforming reference algorithms when tested on a large dataset.

Keywords: Elderly fall detection · Micro electro mechanical system
Inertial measurement unit · Support vector machine
Multi-layer perceptron · K-nearest neighbors

1 Introduction

In recent years, the number of old people is increasing rapidly [1]. One of the problems that often arise is the problem of falls. Moreover, old people would rather stay at home than live in some retirement home [1]. In these risky situations, it is very important to provide adequate interventions for the elderly when a fall occurs. Therefore, many devices have been developed to detect falls automatically. Fall detection devices can be divided into three categories: wearable, ambiance and camera based devices [2,3]. The main drawbacks of ambiance and camera based devices are the expensive hardware costs and the fact that their usage is limited to indoor environments. Moreover, wearable devices commonly use inertial measurement units like accelerometers and gyroscopes as well as magnetometers or a fusion between different sensors in order to capture human movements. Thanks to the rapid development of the micro-electromechanical systems, wearable fall detection devices can be implemented as small, lightweight and low-cost devices [4].

Fall detection algorithms used in the literature can be divided into threshold-based and machine learning-based methods. One of the recent and efficient

© ICST Institute for Computer Sciences, Social Informatics and Telecommunications Engineering 2018
M. U. Ahmed et al. (Eds.): HealthyIoT 2017, LNICST 225, pp. 34–41, 2018.
https://doi.org/10.1007/978-3-319-76213-5_5

threshold-based algorithms is the work by Pierleoni *et al.* [5] where authors designed and implemented a wearable fall detector with four sensors that are accelerometer, gyroscope, magnetometer and barometer. The first three sensors are used to estimate the orientation of the body. This is achieved depending on an efficient quaternion-based and low-computational complexity sensor fusion algorithm namely Madgwick's algorithm [6]. Once the orientation is estimated, it is used to rotate the acceleration vector from the sensor frame into the Earth frame. Then the Earth gravity vector (that is known in the Earth frame) is subtracted from the vertical acceleration component in order to get an initial estimate of the dynamic vertical acceleration of the body. The latter is then fused with the output of the barometer in order to achieve an accurate estimate of the dynamic vertical acceleration. This signal is then analyzed and multiple thresholds are applied in order to detect the fall. This algorithm proves its good performance in a variety of experimental scenarios. However, from the power consumption point of view which is a critical topic in designing a wearable device, using four sensors with a relatively complicated sensor fusion algorithm is not recommended as it affects the battery life considerably. The aforementioned drawbacks motivated researchers to use only a 3-axial accelerometer for capturing the human movements. In the present study, the proposed design of the fall detector is only based on an accelerometer. The total three dimensional acceleration $a = [a_x \ a_y \ a_z]^\mathrm{T}$ measured by the accelerometer is a combination of the body acceleration a_{body} and the Earth gravity field g. It is given as follows [7]:

$$a = K[C_n^b(g + a_{body})] + b + v \tag{1}$$

where K denotes the scale factor matrix, C_n^b denotes the direction cosine matrix that represents the orientation of the navigation frame (frame n) with respect to the body frame (frame b), b represents the bias vector and v represents measurement noise. An interesting recent research by Abdelhedi *et al.* [8] proposed a 3-axial accelerometer-based fall detection system that uses multiple predefined thresholds in order to detect the fall. The sum vector magnitude Σ given by Eq. (2) is used as a characteristic signal that is compared with two predefined amplitude thresholds in order to detect the free fall phase and the impact phase respectively, while the body tilt angle θ defined by Eq. (3) is used to detect the inactivity phase when the impact phase is detected:

$$\Sigma = \sqrt{a_x^2 + a_y^2 + a_z^2} \tag{2}$$

$$\theta = \arctan \sqrt{a_y^2 + a_z^2}/a_x \tag{3}$$

This is achieved by comparing the tilt angle with a predefined threshold also. Although the simplicity of the aforementioned algorithm makes it attractive to be embedded in a wearable fall detector, using constant thresholds leads to a significant amount of false alarms because of the similar behavior of some Activities of Daily Living (ADLs) and falls. One more complicated but more accurate methodology is to use machine learning techniques instead of the pre-defined threshold-based ones. Mezghani *et al.* [9] proposed a fall detection algo-rithm based on Support Vector Machine (SVM). Some statistical features are extracted from the motion signal that is acquired using a 3-axial accelerometer. These features are the mean, the minimum, the maximum, the range and the skewness calculated in a time window of a predefined width (see Fig. 1). Features extracted from a training dataset together with the corresponding ground truth (falls/ADLs) are used to learn the SVM. In the practical application, the on-line extracted features represent the inputs of the trained SVM that in turn makes a binary decision of a fall/ADL event. This algorithm achieved high accuracy in detecting falls. However, the false alarm rate needs to be further reduced.

Performance of fall detectors is evaluated in terms of both the successfulness in detecting falls when they occur and the absence of false alarms when no fall is present. These performance criteria are called the sensitivity and specificity respectively. To satisfy these criteria, an efficient machine learning-based fall detection system is proposed in this paper. Moreover, as the power consumption is a critical issue in designing a wearable device, both the sampling frequency and the hardware complexity are taken into account in the system we propose. Particularly, the motion is captured using the accelerometer only leading to a simple and low power consumption hardware design. In addition, as it is well known, lower sampling frequencies lead to lower power consumption. Conse-quently, the performances of the proposed system as well as the reference ones will be analyzed as a function of the sampling frequency in order to determine the best trade-off between performance and power consumption.

The rest of the paper is organized as follows: Sect. 2 describes the proposed methods while Sect. 3 is devoted to the experimental results and Sect. 4 concludes the paper and states the future work.

2   Methods and Materials

In classical supervised machine learning-based methods, the acquired signals are buffered for a predefined time period (called window) and then described within this window by extracting the signal features. These features are used together with the corresponding ground truth (fall/ADL in our case) to train the machine. In practical application, the features are extracted from the lat-est window and applied to the already trained machine that in turn makes its decision (fall/ADL). The proposed approach is based on supervised machine learning with two main contributions: (1) the efficient extracted features and (2) the novel training strategy. These two contributions as well as the proposed fall detection strategy are discussed in the following sub-sections.

2.1   Features Extraction

The key factor underlying the behavior of the machine learning-based methods is the efficiency in building the features that describe the raw signal. Particu-larly, the features vector is preferred to be as short as possible and as much

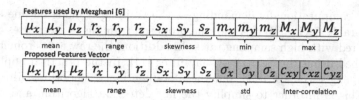

Fig. 1. Proposed features vs. features used by Mezghani [9]

representative of the raw signal as possible. Although the performance of the SVM-based Mezghani algorithm [9] proves to be good, one can note that there is redundancy in the features vector. Particularly, the aforementioned algorithm uses the minimum and maximum values of the signal within the processed time domain and it also uses the range that is the difference between them. Therefore, the components of the features vector are not independent and thus not the best representative ones. To this end, we propose two better representative features than the minimum and maximum statistics. These features are the inter-correlation and standard-deviation. Inter-correlation between the accelerometer components is given by Eq. (4):

$$corr_{(x,y)} = cov(x,y)/(\sigma_x \times \sigma_y) \tag{4}$$

where $cov(x,y)$ is the covariance between x and y axes of the acceleration vector components and σ_x, σ_y are the standard deviations in the processed window. The idea underlying the usage of the inter-correlation feature is its ability to distinguish the activities which involve the movement in one dimension [10]. So, the extracted features employ the inter-correlations between the three components of the acceleration vector expecting a higher sensitivity with a significant reduction in false alarm rate in comparison with the considered reference algorithms that are the SVM-based Mezghani algorithm [9] and the threshold-based Abdelhedi [8] one. In summary, the proposed features vector consists of the mean, the range, the skewness, the standard deviation and the inter-correlation features where the first four features are calculated for all the accelerometer components $(x, y$ and $z)$ and the inter-correlations are calculated between x and y, x and z and y and z respectively. Figure 1 illustrates both the proposed features as well as the features used by Mezghani [9].

2.2 The Proposed Training Strategy

In the literature, most researches (if not all) use the same experimental conditions for both training and practical application. For example, the same sampling frequency for acquiring training data is used in the real application data acquisition. The proposed training strategy is to use optimal training conditions even if they are computationally demanding as the training is made off-line and not on the wearable device. To this end, the proposed training strategy uses training data acquired with high sampling rates. In addition, the raw accelerometer data are smoothed using the Savitzky-Golay filter [11]. In the practical application, lower sampling rates are used and the aforementioned smoothing filter is not applied. This is in order to simplify the fall detection algorithm and to minimize power consumption. The theoretical justification of the proposed strategy is the fact that the objective of machine-learning is to capture the best nonlinear model that separates data classes ideally. That is why this training is better to be done in good conditions even if the practical application conditions are different. Three machine learning methods were explored with the proposed strategy in order to classify the activities into falls or ADLs (binary classification). These methods are the Support Vector Machine (SVM) with a linear kernel function, the K-Nearest Neighbors (KNN) and the Multi-Layer Perceptron (MLP).

2.3   Fall Detection Strategy

In the proposed fall detection strategy, the elderly activity is recorded and continuously buffered in overlapped sliding windows of a predefined width. The features extracted from the last window form the input of the trained machine. When the machine detects a fall, a counter is used to count the successive detections of the same fall. If the aforementioned counter exceeds a predefined threshold, the activity is considered as a fall. This strategy is useful to reduce the amount of false alarms making use of the large overlap between the successive windows. Moreover, as soon as a fall is detected, a beep is generated by the device and a counter is started. This is to give the elderly a capability to cancel the alarm if he/she can recover or if the alarm is just a false one. When the timer exceeds a predefined threshold, an alarm is sent to a medical team (or any authorized person) with the geographical position of the elderly.

3   Experimental Results

The performance of the proposed method is evaluated and compared with the reference SVM-based Mezghani algorithm [9] and the threshold-based Abdelhedi algorithm [8], applying the three following criteria: sensitivity, specificity and accuracy [12]. Experimental analysis is performed using a large reference open dataset, namely Sisfall [13]. In this dataset, the number of activities (falls and ADLs) files exceeds 4510 and are recorded on 37 subjects. All activities were acquired at the sampling frequency $F_s = 200$ Hz. From the aforementioned dataset, 16 ADL types which are the most common in elderly activities were selected for training together with 15 fall types gathered from 12 young subjects and 8 elderly ones. Numerically, the training set consists of 1864 samples

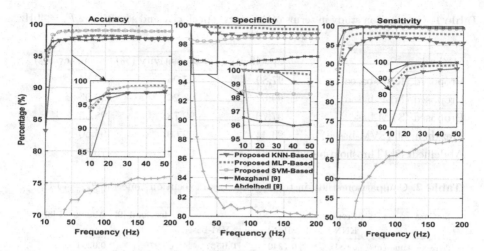

Fig. 2. The proposed KNN, MLP and SVM-based methods vs. the reference algorithms [8,9] in terms of accuracy, specificity and sensitivity for $F_s \in [10, 200]$ Hz

while the testing set consists of 1792 samples. Figure 2 illustrates the preliminary results using the aforementioned performance criteria as functions of sampling frequency. This frequency analysis is achieved by down-sampling the original signals $F_s \in \{200, 190, ..., 10\}$ Hz (without any smoothing). We note from Fig. 2 that the sampling frequencies above 40 Hz are not needed as the performance is approximately constant over this value. This frequency is recommended to be used in the machine learning-based fall detectors as it is the minimal frequency for efficient performance. This result is justified also theoretically as the maximum frequency of human movements is 20 Hz [10]. That is why it is sufficient to acquire data using 40 Hz sampling frequency (Nyquist frequency). We note also from Fig. 2 that the SVM-based proposed method outperforms the reference algorithms in terms of accuracy and specificity over all sampling frequencies whereas it shows approximately the same sensitivity as the SVM-based reference one. Table 1 shows the preliminary numerical results for $F_s = 40$ Hz. As expected, the four machine learning-based methods outperform the threshold-based one. We can note also that the SVM-based proposed method outperforms Mezghani approach [9] in terms of all performance criteria with a significant difference in the specificity, meaning that a lower rate of false alarm could be achieved using our method thanks to the efficient extracted features. Table 2 shows the average execution time of the considered methods. The execution time is comparable for the four machine learning-based methods. Now, if the threshold-based algorithm shows a reduced execution time, it is at the expense of performance quality.

Table 1. Comparison study in terms of accuracy, specificity and sensitivity; $F_s = 40$Hz

Method	Specificity (%)	Sensitivity (%)	Accuracy (%)
Proposed (KNN-based)	97.89	97.06	97.54
Proposed (MLP-based)	99.62	98.26	99.05
Proposed (SVM-based)	97.70	99.73	98.55
Mezghani [9] (SVM-based)	94.44	99.60	96.60
Abdelhedi [8] (Threshold-based)	82.85	54.14	70.87

Table 2. Comparison study in terms of average execution time for $F_s = 40$ Hz

Method	Proposed			Mezghani [9]	Abdelhedi [8]
	KNN-based	MLP-based	SVM-based		
Av. exe. time (ms)	0.6818	0.7240	0.6567	0.6278	0.0254

4   Conclusion

In this paper, an efficient design of a machine learning-based elderly fall detector is proposed. The design takes into account the power consumption issue that is critical in wearable devices. To this end, a single 3-axial accelerometer is used to capture the elderly motion with a sampling frequency of 40 Hz that showed the best trade-off between performance and power consumption. The preliminary results of the proposed system are quite promising. Thanks to the efficient extracted features and the new training procedure, the proposed method outperforms reference algorithms in terms of both sensitivity and specificity throughout the whole range of studied sampling frequencies. The proposed design is under hardware implementation and the performance on hardware will be explored in a future work. In addition, more efficient features would be investigated in order to further reduce the false alarm rate.

Acknowledgments. This publication is supported by the European Union through the European Regional Development Fund (ERDF), the Ministry of Higher Education and Research, the French region of Brittany and Rennes Métropole.

References

1. Bloom, D.E., Boersch-Supan, A., McGee, P., Seike, A.: Population aging: facts, challenges, and responses. Program on the Global Demography of Aging, Massachusetts (2011)
2. Yu, X.: Approaches and principles of fall detection for elderly and patient. In: 10th International Conference on e-Health Networking, Applications and Services (2008)
3. Chaccour, K., Darazi, R., Hassani, A.H., Andrès, E.: From fall detection to fall prevention: a generic classification of fall-related systems. IEEE Sens. J. **17**, 812–822 (2017)

4. Attal, F., Mohammed, S., Dedabrishvili, M., Chamroukhi, F., Oukhellou, L., Amirat, Y.: Physical human activity recognition using wearable sensors. Sensors **15**, 31314–31338 (2015)
5. Pierleoni, P., Belli, A., Maurizi, L., Palma, L., Pernini, L., Paniccia, M., Valenti, S.: A wearable fall detector for elderly people based on AHRS and barometric sensor. IEEE Sens. J. **16**, 6733–6744 (2016)
6. Madgwick, S.O.H., Harrison, A.J.L., Vaidyanathan, R.: Estimation of IMU and MARG orientation using a gradient descent algorithm. In: IEEE International Conference on Rehabilitation Robotics, Zurich, Switzerland (2011)
7. Sabatini, A.M.: Quaternion-based extended Kalman filter for determining orientation by inertial and magnetic sensing. IEEE Trans. Biomed. Eng. **53**(7), 1346–1356 (2006)
8. Abdelhedi, S., Bourguiba, R., Mouine, J., Baklouti, M.: Development of a two-threshold-based fall detection algorithm for elderly health monitoring. In: IEEE 10th International Conference on Research Challenges in Information Science (RCIS), Grenoble, France (2016)
9. Mezghani, N., Ouakrim, Y., Islam, M.R., Yared, R., Abdulrazak, B.: Context aware adaptable approach for fall detection bases on smart textile. In: IEEE International Conference on Biomedical & Health Informatics (BHI), Orlando, USA (2017)
10. Cleland, I., Kikhia, B., Nugent, C., Boytsov, A., Hallberg, J., Synnes, K., McClean, S., Finlay, D.: Optimal placement of accelerometers for the detection of everyday activities. Sensors **13**, 9183–9200 (2013)
11. Savitzky, A., Golay, M.J.E.: Smoothing and differentiation of data by simplified least squares procedures. Anal. Chem. **36**(8), 1627–1639 (1964)
12. Casilari, E., Luque, R., Morón, M.J.: Analysis of android device-based solutions for fall detection. Sensors **15**, 17827–17894 (2015)
13. Sucerquia, A., López, J.D., Vargas-Bonilla, J.F.: SisFall: a fall and movement dataset. Sensors **17**, 198 (2017)

Characterization of Home-Acquired Blood Pressure Time Series Using Multiscale Entropy for Patients Treated Against Kidney Cancer

Antoine Jamin[1](✉), Jean-Baptiste Fasquel[1], Anne Humeau-Heurtier[1], Pierre Abraham[2], Georges Leftheriotis[3], and Samir Henni[1,2]

[1] LARIS, Université d'Angers, 62 Avenue Notre-Dame du Lac, 49000 Angers, France
antjamin@etud.univ-angers.fr
[2] Vascular Departement and MITOVASC, University Hospital Center of Angers, Angers, France
[3] Vascular Departement, University Hospital Center of Nice, Nice, France

Abstract. This study deals with the telemonitoring, with a connected tensiometer, of 16 patients treated for a kidney cancer. Each one of these patients recorded his/her blood pressure at home during 63 days and the data was sent to his/her medical doctor. At the same time they were treated with antihypertensive medication when necessary. In this work, our goal was to analyze the complexity of the blood pressure time series. For this purpose, we proposed to use the refined composite multiscale entropy (RCMSE) measures. Our results show that the patterns of RCMSE through temporal scales evolve with the antihypertensive medication. The later might therefore have an impact on home-acquired blood pressure complexity. RCMSE could therefore be an interesting information theory-based tool to study home-acquired physiological data.

Keywords: Telemonitoring · Connected tensiometer
Blood pressure · Time series · Multiscale entropy · Clustering
Irregularity · Complexity

1 Introduction

Kidney cancer is the 12th kind of cancer in terms of frequency in the world. It represents 338,000 new cases diagnosed in 2012 [1]. It can be treated by a VEGF[1] chemotherapy that consists in eliminating the capillaries of the tumor. However such a treatment can lead to blood pressure increases. This is why antihypertensive medication are often given to the patients. Our work deals with patients treated against a kidney cancer using a VEGF chemotherapy. During the treatment, patients recorded their blood pressure once a day at home using a

---

[1] Vascular Endothelial Growth Factor.

© ICST Institute for Computer Sciences, Social Informatics and Telecommunications Engineering 2018
M. U. Ahmed et al. (Eds.): HealthyIoT 2017, LNICST 225, pp. 42–47, 2018.
https://doi.org/10.1007/978-3-319-76213-5_6

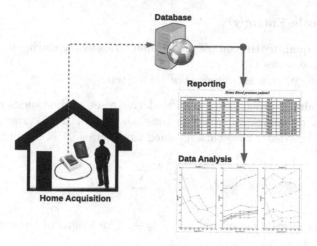

Fig. 1. Project overview

connected tensiometer (see Fig. 1). Such an IoT-based sensor [2,3] facilitates the following of blood pressure increases. Our goal herein is to study, with the refined composite multiscale entropy (RCMSE), the complexity of the blood pressure time series.

RCMSE is an improved version of the multiscale entropy (MSE). MSE relies on the sample entropy algorithm and on a coarse-graining procedure to study irregularity of time series at different time scales [4].

The paper is organized as follows: the MSE and RCMSE algorithms and the measurement procedure are introduced in Sect. 2. Our results are then detailed and discussed in Sect. 3. The paper ends with a Conclusion.

2   Materials and Methods

2.1   Sample Entropy

Pincus proposed to quantify the irregularity of time series with approximate entropy (ApEn) [5]. To overcome the limitation of ApEn, sample entropy has later been introduced [6]. Sample entropy is a conditional probability measure that quantifies the likelihood that a sequence of m consecutive data points – that matches another sequence of the same length – will still match the other sequence when their length is increased by one sample $(m+1)$ [4]. Sample entropy is computed as:

$$SampEn(m, r, N) = -\ln \frac{A^m(r)}{B^m(r)}, \tag{1}$$

where r is the tolerance, m is the sample length, $A^m(r)$ and $B^m(r)$ are, respectively, the probability that two sequences will match for $m + 1$ and m points.

2.2   Multiscale Entropy

MSE allows to quantify the complexity of time series by measuring its irregularity at different time scales [4,6].

The MSE algorithm is composed of three steps [7,8]

1. a coarse-graining procedure is used to derive a set of time series representing the system dynamics on different time scales. For a monovariate discrete signal x of length N, the coarse-grained time series y^τ is computed as:

$$y_j^{(\tau)} = \frac{1}{\tau} \sum_{i=(j-1)\tau+1}^{j\tau} x_i, \tag{2}$$

   where τ is the scale factor and $1 \leqslant j \leqslant \frac{N}{\tau}$. The length of the coarse-grained time series is N/τ.
2. computation of the sample entropy for each coarse-grained times series.
3. plot of the sample entropy for each time scale τ.

2.3   Refined Composite Multiscale Entropy

MSE generates some undefined values for short time series [9]. When large scale factors τ are used, the coarse-grained time series may have a small number of samples. This may lead to undefined sample entropy values. This is why RCMSE has been introduced [9].

In RCMSE, the coarse-grained signal $y_k^{(\tau)}$ is computed for different values of a parameter k:

$$y_{k,j}^{(\tau)} = \frac{1}{\tau} \sum_{i=(j-1)\tau+k}^{j\tau+k-1} x_i, \tag{3}$$

where τ is the scale factor, x is the original signal, $1 \leqslant j \leqslant \frac{N}{\tau}$ and $1 \leqslant k \leqslant \tau$.

The RCMSE at scale τ is calculated using the following formulation:

$$RCMSE(x, \tau, m, r) = -\ln \frac{\sum_{k=1}^{\tau} n_{k,\tau}^{m+1}}{\sum_{k=1}^{\tau} n_{k,\tau}^{m}}, \tag{4}$$

where r is the tolerance, m is the sample length, $n_{k,\tau}^{m+1}$ and $n_{k,\tau}^{m}$ are the number of matched vector pairs (computed on $y_k^{(\tau)}$) for $m+1$ and m, respectively.

2.4   Measurement Procedure

The study was conducted on 16 patients (5 women, 11 men; 171 cm $\pm$ 9 cm; 87 kg $\pm$ 29 kg; 62 years $\pm$ 8 years). The 16 patients were daily monitored, during 63 days, using a connected tensiometer (Tel-O-Graph®, I.E.M. GmbH). Each recorded time series (Systolic Blood Pressure (SBP) and Diastolic Blood Pressure (DBP) time series) had therefore 63 samples. In our work, $MBP(k)$

processed by RCMSE was defined as $MBP(k) = (SBP(k) + 2 \times DBP(k))/3$, $1 \leqslant k \leqslant 63$, where $SBP(k)$ is the systolic blood pressure at day k, $DBP(k)$ is the diastolic blood pressure at day k and $MBP(k)$ is the mean blood pressure at day k.

2.5   Parameters Used

To compute RCMSE, 3 parameters have to be set: m, r, and τ. It has been recommended that, to compute the sample entropy, the time series length has to be between 10^m and 20^m [6]. Our data have 63 samples. We therefore have chosen $m = 1$ and time scale $\tau \leqslant 5$. Moreover, we have chosen $r = 0.15 \times \sigma$ (where σ is the standard deviation of time series at scale factor $\tau = 1$) [8].

3   Results and Discussion

Figure 2 presents three examples of MBP time series. Figure 3 shows the corresponding RCMSE curves. By analyzing all the time series we observe 3 kinds of RCMSE patterns: global decreasing sample entropy with scales (cluster 1), global increasing sample entropy with scales (cluster 2), and non-monotonic sample entropy values with scales (cluster 3); see Fig. 4.

If sample entropy increases with scales, this means that the signal contains complex structures across multiple scales. If the sample entropy decreases with scales, this means that the signal has information only on the shortest scale (similarly to white noise [8]). In the undetermined case, no definite conclusion can be drawn.

We can observe that the signals of cluster 1 are similar to RCMSE of a white noise: the signal irregularity decreases with scale. Cluster 2 corresponds to an increase of the signal irregularity with scales. Cluster 3 corresponds to an intermediate situation.

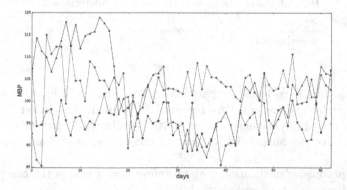

Fig. 2. Representative signals for each cluster (cluster 1: red — cluster 2: blue — cluster 3: green). (Color figure online)

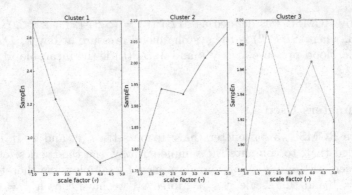

Fig. 3. RCMSE and clusters of representative signals shown in Fig. 2.

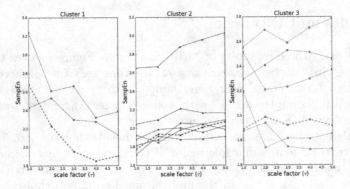

Fig. 4. RCMSE and clusters. Original signals leading to dotted RCMSE are represented in Fig. 2

Table 1. Clusters, RCMSE and #medication

Cluster	Cluster 1	Cluster 2	Cluster 3
RCMSE shape	Decrease	Increase	Undetermined
#patients	3	7	6
#medication	1	2	3

These clusters have been compared with the number of hypertensive medication taken by the patients. As reported in Table 1, for cluster 1, patients received only 1 antihypertensive treatment. For cluster 2, patients received 2 antihypertensive treatments. For cluster 3, patients received 3 antihypertensive treatments.

Anti-hypertensive medication may therefore play a role in the complexity of mean blood pressure time series.

4   Conclusion

In this work we studied the complexity of blood pressure time series with RCMSE. Further work is needed to apply the RCMSE algorithm on much more data. However, our work shows that antihypertensive medication might have an influence on mean blood pressure complexity. Our study shows that the complexity of data extracted by connected devices may be interesting for physiological purposes. Now, RCMSE could be applied to other IoT-based physiological time series. The next step of our work will consist in identifying patient profiles in order to personalize the telemonitoring.

References

1. World Cancer Research Fund International, May 2017. http://www.wcrf.org
2. Yin, Y., Zeng, Y., Chen, X., Fan, Y.: The internet of things in healthcare: an overview. J. Ind. Inform. Integr. **1**, 3–13 (2016)
3. Islam, S.M.R., Kwak, D., Kabir, M.H., Hossain, M., Kwak, K.S.: The Internet of Things for health care: a comprehensive survey. IEEE Access **3**, 678–708 (2015)
4. Humeau-Heurtier, A.: The multiscale entropy algorithm and its variants: a review. Entropy **17**, 3110–3123 (2015)
5. Pincus, S.M.: Approximate entropy as a measure of system complexity. Proc. Natl. Acad. Sci. **88**, 2297–2301 (1991)
6. Richman, J.S., Moorman, J.R.: Physiological time-series analysis using approximate entropy and sample entropy. Am. J. Physiol. Heart Circulatory Physiol. **278**, H2039–H2049 (2000)
7. Costa, M., Goldberger, A.L., Peng, C.-K.: Multiscale entropy analysis of complex physiologic time series. Phys. Rev. Lett. **89**, 068102 (2002)
8. Costa, M., Goldberger, A.L., Peng, C.-K.: Multiscale entropy analysis of biological signals. Phys. Rev. E **71**, 021906 (2005)
9. Wu, S.-D., Wu, C.-W., Lin, S.-G., Lee, K.-Y., Peng, C.-K.: Analysis of complex time series using refined composite multiscale entropy. Phys. Lett. A **378**, 1369–1374 (2014)

A Heterogeneous IoT-Based Architecture for Remote Monitoring of Physiological and Environmental Parameters

Gordana Gardašević[1]([✉]) [iD], Hossein Fotouhi[2], Ivan Tomasic[2],
Maryam Vahabi[2], Mats Björkman[2], and Maria Lindén[2]

[1] Faculty of Electrical Engineering, University of Banja Luka, Banja Luka,
Bosnia and Herzegovina
gordana.gardasevic@etf.unibl.org
[2] Mälardalen University, Västerås, Sweden
{hossein.fotouhi,ivan.tomasic,maryam.vahabi,mats.bjorkman,
maria.linden}@mdh.se

Abstract. A heterogeneous Internet of Things (IoT) architecture for remote health monitoring (RHM) is proposed, that employs Bluetooth and IEEE 802.15.4 wireless connectivity. The RHM system encompasses Shimmer physiological sensors with Bluetooth radio, and OpenMote environmental sensors with IEEE 802.15.4 radio. This system architecture collects measurements in a relational database in a local server to implement a Fog node for fast data analysis as well as in a remote server in the Cloud.

Keywords: Internet of Things · Remote health monitoring · WSN
IEEE 802.15.4e · TSCH · 6TiSCH · OpenMote · OpenWSN
Shimmer

1 Introduction

Wireless Sensors Networks (WSNs) are considered as one of the key Internet of Things (IoT) technologies, and are widely used in various application areas such as environmental and structural monitoring systems, industrial automation, healthcare systems, traffic management and logistics, and public safety. An efficient IoT healthcare system aims to provide a remote health monitoring (RHM) of a patient health status in real-time, the prevention of critical patient conditions, life quality improvement of the elderly through the smart environment, medical and drugs' database administration, and wellbeing services. The IoT smart sensors for healthcare enable accurately measuring, monitoring and analyzing a variety of vital health status indicators, such as heart rate, ECG, blood pressure, blood glucose levels and oxygen saturation. These sensors are being assigned a unique IPv6 address and integrated in the IPv6 IoT environment. Sensor readings are then collected and transferred to the IP end-devices or to the Cloud [1].

© ICST Institute for Computer Sciences, Social Informatics and Telecommunications Engineering 2018
M. U. Ahmed et al. (Eds.): HealthyIoT 2017, LNICST 225, pp. 48–53, 2018.
https://doi.org/10.1007/978-3-319-76213-5_7

Recently, the IEEE 802.15.4e standard has been proposed as a MAC amendment to the existing IEEE 802.15.4-2011 standard [2]. The specific mode, called Time Synchronized Channel Hopping (TSCH), significantly increases robustness against external interference and multipath fading while running on IEEE 802.15.4 hardware. TSCH is particularly efficient in providing ultra low-power operation. Defining IPv6 over the TSCH mode of IEEE 802.15.4e (6TiSCH) is a key to enable further adoption of IPv6 in industrial and healthcare IoT domains [3]. Therefore, we propose the use of IoT platform based on OpenMote hardware devices and OpenWSN operating system, both rooted in the new 6TiSCH standard. We believe that the use of this IoT platform in healthcare field can bring many benefits, particularly in terms of reliability and security.

Previously, Archip et al. [4] have investigated the integration of Medlab's physiological sensor boards [5] with Zolteria Z1 [6] board featuring IEEE 802.15.4. However, Mathur et al. [7] employed OpenMote with Contiki in their proposed IoT solution, but neglecting physiological sensors. In our recent work [8] we have investigated the inclusion of relational databases in the architecture for RHM and assumed only Bluetooth connection to physiological sensors. Here we extend that architectural concept by including IEEE 802.15.4 radio, environmental parameters from OpenMote devices running OpenWSN, as well as considering the concept of Fog and Cloud as local and remote storage units.

The structure of the paper is as follows. Section 2 gives an overview on the OpenWSN protocol stack implementation based on 6TiSCH architecture. The details on the system's architecture and components are provided in Sect. 3. Finally, we conclude the paper with indicating future directions in Sect. 4.

2   OpenWSN Protocol Stack

The OpenWSN is a recently released open-source implementation of a fully standard-based protocol stack for IoT capillary networks, rooted in the TSCH standard – see Fig. 1 [9]. The IEEE 802.15.4e TSCH standard replaces the traditional MAC protocol without changing the underlying IEEE 802.15.4 physical layer. Due to its time synchronization and channel hopping, TSCH enables ultra-low power and highly reliable mesh networks. The logical link layer (uRES) is the partial implementation of the IETF 6TiSCH standard. The 6LoWPAN layer enables the integration of IPv6 protocol in low data rate WPANs. The RPL is the routing protocol responsible for packet forwarding between nodes in multi-hop networks. At the transport layer, UDP protocol is used due to its lightweight implementation. CoAP application layer simplifies Web integration and interactive communication between application end-points. The OpenVisualizer (OV) is a Python-based debugging and visualization program in OpenWSN.

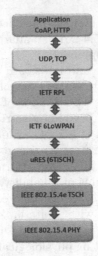

Fig. 1. OpenWSN protocol stack.

3   IoT Healthcare Architecture

We propose the initial framework for IoT platform based on Bluetooth and IEEE 802.15.4 wireless connectivity as illustrated in Fig. 2. The implementation of 6TiSCH protocol stack in RHM field brings many benefits, and is also foreseen as a possible reference for Healthcare 4.0 initiative. Sensors attached to the patients' body sample raw data, and send it to the final destination (local server in the Fog or remote server in the Cloud). A PC acts as a Gateway by supporting both Bluetooth and IEEE 802.15.4 radios. To provide the reliable and secure transmission, the OpenMote device selects the best data path based on the link quality metrics (e.g., LQI, RSSI and ETX) or network metrics (e.g., remaining energy, end-to-end delay, throughput, and traffic level). This prevents packet collisions and/or battery depletion that leads to data losses. Due to scheduled and synchronized transmission, 6TiSCH network provides end-to-end resource reservations and trafic flow isolation, thus enabling a secure acquisition of heterogeneous data.

3.1   System Components

The proposed platform for IoT RHM is the modification of the system architecture presented in [8]. The modified architecture enables data collection from multiple sensors (both on-body and environmental) in order to process and extract useful information about current state of the patient, and also about environment in which a patients resides. We use the OpenMote devices for environmental parameter monitoring, whereas Shimmers provide physiological parameters. Web-based real-time monitoring makes it very easy to identify each device and to obtain sensor values – see Fig. 3.

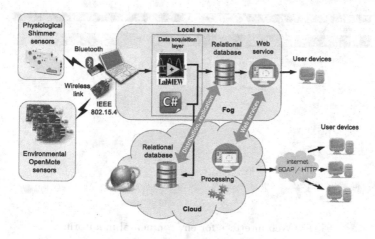

Fig. 2. The system architecture.

Wireless sensors. Shimmer is a wireless sensor platform for RHM applications [10]. Each Shimmer3 ECG/EMG unit provides an inertial measurement unit (IMU) including accelerometer, gyroscope, and magnetometer, as well as ECG unit, which additionally provides 3 ECG leads (limb leads plus one precordial lead). The acquired signals can be stored locally on the device or streamed via Bluetooth. The maximal sampling frequency of the Shimmer3 is 8 kHz. With respect to energy consumption, according to measurements presented in [11], Shimmer sensor with ECG module runs for almost 10 h on its built-in battery, while sending ECG data continuously on the Bluetooth wireless link.

The OpenMote device is a representative of new generation open-hardware platforms [12]. The OpenMote-CC2538 is based on TI CC2538 SoC functionalities, thus combining the 32-bit ARM Cortex-M3 MCU with the IEEE 802.15.4 transceiver. The OpenMote platform has 32 KB of RAM and 512 KB of flash memory, and supports several peripherals, such as GPIOs, ADC, I2C, SPI, UART, timer modules, and AES/RSA Encryption Engine. OpenMote has 3 digital sensors (temperature/humidity, light, accelerometer). The accelerometer may be used to track the movements (activity/inactivity sensing, free fall detection). The OpenMote has a battery supply, so it can be displaced easily within the monitored area. By careful separation of Bluetooth and OpenMote devices, the coexistence without interference can be achieved. The OpenMote indoor transmission range is around 50 m, and in outdoor environments is around 200 m. In this way, the OpenMote can extend current Shimmer capabilities (Bluetooth radio), and thus providing monitoring for bigger area.

Data acquisition layer. The data acquisition layer involves gathering signals from sensor nodes and preparing them for storage, analysis and presentation. Shimmer platform includes three interfaces for data acquisition implemented in MATLAB, LabView and C#.NET, whereas for the OpenMote, OpenWSN has integrated data acquisition and makes the data available on the local web server

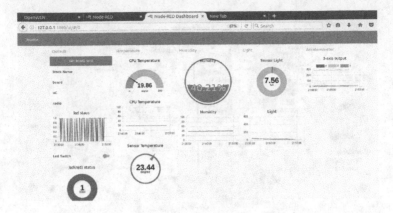

Fig. 3. Web-interface for environmental monitoring.

or Cloud. The data can be inserted in the database immediately upon arrival, either by taking values from the web service (applicable for both sensors) or using the interfaces (Shimmer only).

Database. In our previous work, we presented a relational database structure for RHM [8], which can handle physiological, movement and environmental data, the data about questionnaires and related answers, as well as the general data about patients and system users. In general, any custom relational database can be used. Alternatively to using relational databases it is also possible to store the data in files only or to use NoSQL databases that can, in the same way as relational database, reside on the local server (Fog node) and/or in the Cloud.

Web service and web interface. Local or remote web services can provide data to multiple web interfaces (clients) at a time. The interface is organized as a number of configurable and adjustable graphs that present the data continuously – see Fig. 3. A historical view has also been implemented. This web structure was chosen for the presentational layer instead of a desktop application as in this way the presentational layer is platform independent and easily accessible.

Cloud. The Cloud is a very useful platform for RHM since it can store the acquired measurements, apply already available processing abilities to the data (e.g. [13, 14]), and make the data available to the clients. The data can be fed to the database in a Cloud directly from the data acquisition layer, or the databases in the Cloud can be an automatic replica of the local database. An additional interesting possibility is to use distributed relational databases in which case a part of the database can be kept locally, whereas another part can reside in the Cloud – see Fig. 2. Similarly, the web service in the Cloud can expose the data from the Cloud database, but it can also communicate through web protocols (REST, SOAP, MQTT) to the web service on the local server.

4   Conclusion

This paper presents the preliminary design of a heterogeneous RHM system by considering both physiological and environmental sensors empowered with Bluetooth and IEEE 802.15.4 radios. The hardware and software heterogeneity brings many challenges that incorporates with reliable and secure wireless data communication, while providing smart data analysis at different levels. In the future, we will perform extensive experiments to evaluate the quality of service of the system in various environmental and network conditions.

Acknowledgment. We would like to acknowledge the funding from the Swedish Knowledge Foundation (KKS) throughout research profile Embedded Sensor System for Health (ESS-H), and the distributed environments E-care@home. G. Gardašević acknowledges financial support by EUROWEB+ program. I. Tomasic additionally acknowledges the funding by KKS project CCOPD (reference number: 20160029).

References

1. Gardašević, G., Veletić, M., Maletić, N., Vasiljević, D., Radusinović, I., Tomović, S., Radonjić, M.: The IoT architectural framework, design issues and application domains. Wirel. Pers. Commun. **92**(1), 127–148 (2017)
2. IEEE Standard for Local and Metropolitan Area Networks - Part 15.4: Low-Rate Wireless Personal Area Networks (LR-WPANs) Amendment 1: MAC sublayer (2012)
3. IPv6 over the TSCH mode of IEEE 802.15.4e (6TiSCH). https://datatracker.ietf.org/wg/6tisch/documents/. Accessed 05 July 2017
4. Archip, A., Botezatu, N., Serban, E., Herghelegiu, P.C., Zală, A.: An IoT based system for remote patient monitoring. In: ICCC, pp. 1–6 (2016)
5. Modules for patient monitors. http://www.medlab-gmbh.de/english/modules/index.html. Accessed 05 July 2017
6. RE-Mote. http://zolertia.io/product/hardware/re-mote. Accessed 05 July 2017
7. Mathur, A., Newe, T., Elgenaidi, W., Rao, M., Dooly, G., Toal, D.: A secure end-to-end IoT solution. Sens. Actuators A Phys. **263**, 291–299 (2017)
8. Tomasic, I., Petrovic, N., Fotouhi, H., Lindén, M., Björkman, M.: Data flow and collection for remote patients monitoring: from wireless sensors through a relational database to a web interface in real time. In: Eskola, H., Väisänen, O., Viik, J., Hyttinen, J. (eds.) EMBEC 2017, NBC 2017. IFMBE, vol. 65, pp. 89–92. Springer, Singapore (2017). https://doi.org/10.1007/978-981-10-5122-7_23
9. OpenWSN project. http://www.openwsn.org/. Accessed 07 July 2017
10. Shimmer Technology. Shimmer Discovery in Motion (2017). Accessed 1 Feb 2017
11. Benferhat, D., Guidec, F., Quinton, P.: Cardiac monitoring of marathon runners using disruption-tolerant wireless sensors. In: Bravo, J., López-de-Ipiña, D., Moya, F. (eds.) UCAmI 2012. LNCS, vol. 7656, pp. 395–402. Springer, Heidelberg (2012). https://doi.org/10.1007/978-3-642-35377-2_55
12. OpenMote platform. http://www.openmote.com/. Accessed 07 July 2017
13. Li, Y., Guo, L., Guo, Y.: Enabling health monitoring as a service in the cloud. In: 2014 IEEE/ACM 7th International Conference on Utility and Cloud Computing, pp. 127–136 (2014)
14. Bamarouf, F., Crandell, C., Tsuyuki, S., Sanchez, J., Lu, Y.: Cloud-based real-time heart monitoring and ECG signal processing. In: IEEE SENSORS, pp. 1–3 (2016)

An RFID Based Activity of Daily Living
for Elderly with Alzheimer's

Muhammad Wasim Raad$^{(\boxtimes)}$, Tarek Sheltami,
Mohamed Abdelmonem Soliman, and Muntadar Alrashed

Computer Engineering Department, King Fahd University of Petroleum
and Minerals, Dhahran 31261, Saudi Arabia
{raad, tarek, s201381570, s201139210}@kfupm.edu.sa

Abstract. With the proliferation of emerging technologies such as Internet of Things (IOT) and Radio Frequency identification (RFID), it is possible to collect massive amount of data for localization and tracking of people within commercial buildings & smart homes. In this paper we present the design, implementation and testing of an RFID system for monitoring the wandering about of an Elderly with Alzheimer's at home. The novelty of the algorithm presented lies in its simplicity to detect the motion of elderly from one room to another for monitoring activity of daily living (ADL) and sending alert in case of an onset of emergency without the need for using massive sensors. The system was tested successfully in the lab and achieved an efficiency of 88%.

Keywords: IOT · RFID · Indoor localization · RSSI · ADL

1 Introduction

Alzheimer's is one of the most common diseases among the elderly. One of its most notorious symptoms is unawareness of their location. Thus, they are usually kept under constant observation by a nurse to make sure they do not put them self into harm's way. Tracking people's movement in the home is an essential requirement in many occupant-oriented smart home applications such as elderly monitoring, activity recognition. Knowing the Elderly's room location is vital in inferring their activity of daily living (ADL)s. The aim of this project is to propose an RFID-based localization system to reduce the health and safety of patients with short-term memory loss. In the past few years, Radio frequency identification (RFID) technology related applications has become more demanded than ever. The reason is that the implementation of an RFID system has a relatively low cost compared with any other alternatives. One of the most Known RFID based applications is indoor localization which will be utilized by us. Any RFID system consists of two main components. A reader connected with an antenna and many tags with unique serial number for each. The reader is responsible of identifying any tag within a specific zone with the help of the antenna and depending on the type of the tags used. For example, passive tags will provide a limited detection range while the active tags, which has its own internal power source to keep to its RF communication circuit working on continuous manner, will provide much wider range compared with passive tags. By analyzing data obtained by the RFID system, we will

© ICST Institute for Computer Sciences, Social Informatics and Telecommunications Engineering 2018
M. U. Ahmed et al. (Eds.): HealthyIoT 2017, LNICST 225, pp. 54–61, 2018.
https://doi.org/10.1007/978-3-319-76213-5_8

be able to achieve our localization system. Our basic approach is to identify the room location of each patient by monitoring the doorways between the rooms, and by utilizing RFID system to confirm the crossing process, we can determine the new room location [1–4]. In addition to that, Internet of things (IOT) has played a vital role recently particularly for healthcare. The internet of things can be described as connecting everyday objects like smart phones, internet TVs, sensors and actuators to the internet where the devices are intelligently linked together enabling new forms of communication between things and people. It is envisioned that billions of physical things or objects will be outfitted with different kind of sensors and actuators and connected to the internet via heterogeneous networks enabled by technologies such as embedded sensing, RFID and wireless sensor networks. The reliance of healthcare on IOT is increasing to improve access to care, increase the quality of care and most importantly reduce the cost of care [5, 6]. Section 2 constitutes overview of overall proposed system including RSSI scanning algorithms. Section 3 constitutes the experimental results. The novelty of the proposed system compared to existing localization & tracking systems for activity of daily living lies in the fact that it only tracks the direction of motion of the elderly from one room to another and detecting his/her inactivity without the need to employ massive sensors. For the sake of simplifying the design we assumed a home consisting of two rooms only.

2 Overview

Our indoor localization system has four main components:

1. Mat Pressure Sensor
2. Reader and Antennas
3. RFID Tags
4. Crossing Detection Algorithms

All of these components are integrated together to provide the desired system efficiency.

2.1 Layout

1. *Pressure Mat Sensors:* In order to reduce the error and enhance the system efficiency, an extra level of detection is implemented. By placing two pressure mat sensors on both sides on the doorway, we will be able to detect when someone is trying to enter or leave a specific room. In case there is an attempt to cross the door, the system will be informed and consequently the reader will be triggered to initiate the electromagnetic radiation to energize the tags and thus collecting the required data to determine the patient room location. To monitor doorway crossings, we create two RF sensing zones initiated by two separate antennas, one on each side of the doorway. See Figs. 2 and 3. By knowing which of the two sensing zones of the

doorway was crossed first, the direction of motion can be determined. To be detected by the RF doormats, the Elderly must wear passive RFID bracelets around the ankles. Ankles are always at a consistent orientation and distance from the floor when walking, thereby converting a 3D positioning problem to 2D presence/absence decision. Moreover, in order to prevent repetitive pulses generated from the pressure mat sensors when pressed, a timing circuit is connecting the sensors to the reader's general purpose input/output (GPIO). The timing circuit utilizes 555 Timer IC to produce a constant output DC voltage of 1–15 V for about 20 s, and it will remain constant even if the mat is pressed again during the 20 s (See Fig. 1).

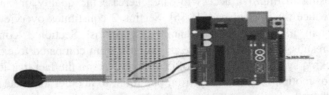

Fig. 1. Hardware layout

2. *Reader and Antennas:* An UHF (ultra-high frequency) frequency range is used for two Antennas with specific configurations controlled by a Sirit reader. The antennas are used to create two separated sensing zones, one of the zones should cover one side of the doorway, the other one will cover the other side, and both of them will overlap at the doorway (see Fig. 2). Both antennas work in the frequency range of 865–870 MHz. the coverage area of each zone are as shown above and has the following measures:

   - Width of the zone greater ranges from 0.5 to 0.7 m.
   - Length of the zone greater than width of doorway.
   Coverage area is controlled by changing the conducted power to antenna and thus, the power generated by the backscattering signal will vary resulting in different readings. See Fig. 2.

3. *RFID Tags:* The major requirements in the tags that are needed in our indoor localization system are to be user friendly, to have reasonable cost and efficiency. These requirements have led us to utilize passive RFID tag attached to an ankle bracelet. The tags used should be compatible with the UHF antennas mentioned above.

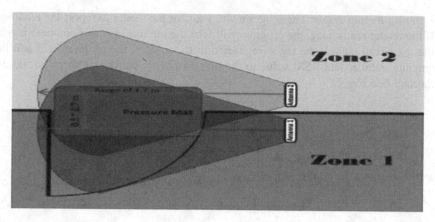

Fig. 2. Layout of the zone based RFID tracking of the elderly through doorway.

2.2   Algorithm

To detect precisely when an Elderly crosses a doorway, the anklet readings are processed by converting the anklet readings (RSSI) into clusters of possible doorway crossing events. A doorway crossing is detected if there are consecutive sets of readings from both of the detection zones of a doorway. The scan algorithm groups the raw RFID data from the sensing zones in each doorway into clusters based on their timestamp. See Fig. 4. There are three parts of the algorithm that composes the system; they are, in chronological order:

1. *Initiating the scan:* The event listener will listen for an event from the reader (when the elderly steps on the Matt situated in the doorway, and connected to Arduino microcontroller). Based on this, the program will retrieve the registered tags from Patient Database and will initialize two kind of array: the first array (i.e. TagAvg) will be used to register Received Signal Strength Indicator (RSSI) for each tag per antenna during the scan period.
2. *Determining the location of the tag (patient):* A thread will wait for scan from the reader (the reader will generate scan_complete_event when it's finished scanning). Then, the program will calculate the average RSSI reading per tag based on the values from first array (i.e. TagAvg). If the obtained average of RSSI for the tag is not equal to zero, it will be added to the second array (i.e. taglog). Initially, a DBscane filter on MatLab was used, but its results proved to be inefficient because the filter extremely smoothed the differences between subsequent RSSI readings of both antennas, which made the timestamps of the strongest readings of both antennas almost the same, thus it couldn't determine which antenna read its max RSSI first. Thus, it was replaced with a simple max filter on java that proved to be much more efficient, this most likely due the setup being efficient and producing already smooth and distinct reading. See Fig. 6 for Java code for reading RSSI.

3. *Filtering the tag reads:* The program will wait for the reader to report tag readings. If the reader reads a tag, the program will take the tag readings and compare it with the registered tags. If the tag is registered in the system, the program will add the antenna number and RSSI value to the first array (i.e. tagAvg). Otherwise, ignore the tag. See Fig. 5.

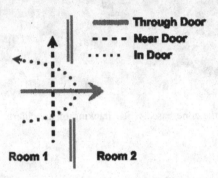

Fig. 3. RF sensing zones on both sides of doorway to determine direction of motion of elderly

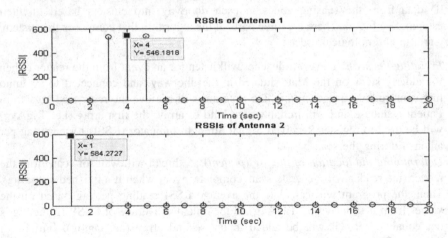

Fig. 4. Temporally sequenced raw data stream of RSSI data reads in 20 s frame from both sides of the doorway

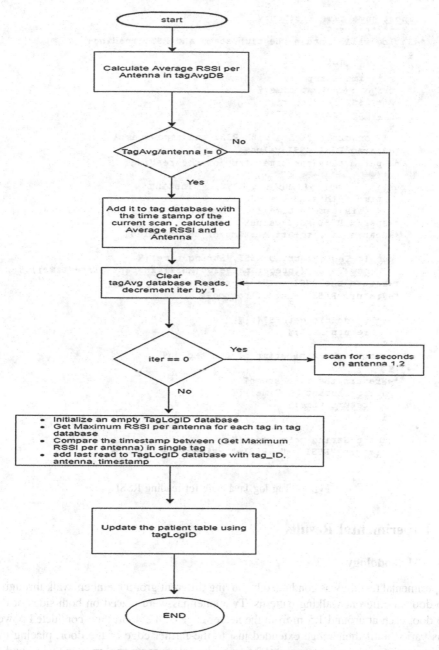

Fig. 5. RFID tag Scan & RSSI filtering Algorithm.

```
import java.time.Instant;
/**************
*→TagLog will contain the time stamp and RSSI reading

public class TagLog {
    /** time stamp **/
    private Instant time;
    /** RSSI reading **/
    private double RSSI;

      **Construct TagLog with RSSI and time stamp
    *→@param RSSI RSSI value
    *→@param time the time stamp of the reading
    */
    public  TagLog(double   RSSI,   Instant
        time){ this.RSSI = RSSI;
          this.time = time;
    *→@param RSSI RSSI value
    *→@param time the time stamp of the reading
    */
    public TagLog(String RSSI, String time){
        new TagLog(Integer.parseInt(RSSI),Instant.parse(time));
    *→return the RSSI value of the tag
    *→@return RSSI value of tagLog
    */
    public double getRSSI(){
        return RSSI;
    }
    *→return the time stamp of the taglog
*  →  
    *→@return the time stamp
    public Instant getTime(){
        return time;
    }

    public String toString(){
        return("RSSI = " +RSSI+", time = "+ time);
    }
```

Fig. 6. Tag log Java code for reading RSSI

3 Experimental Results

3.1 Methodology

Experimental testing was conducted by having different group members walk through a lab door in different walking patterns. Two antennas were placed on both sides of the lab door each at around 1.5 m from the nearer edge of the door, their conducted power was varied until their range extended just to the farther edge of the door, placing the farthest point of the range at around 2.5 m as the antennas were placed on the ground at a right angle and 1 m away from each other. The antennas were also separated by two layers of aluminum foil in order to avoid interference (see Fig. 2). As soon as the Sirit RFID reader was initiated, it would scan 40 times for the duration of 20 s (2 scans/s).

3.2 Results

The system was tested in the RFID lab of King Fahd University of Petroleum and Minerals, and achieved an overall efficiency of 88% after 68 trials; about 50% of the failed trials were due to body shadowing (the tag was too close to the skin or was on the farther side of the farther leg from the antennas), 37.5% was due to hesitant walking patterns (going back and forth between the two zones several times during the scanning period), and 12.5% was due to setup errors (an antenna displaced or conducted power not adjusted). The *Patient checker, part of the algorithm, is* responsible for checking a patient's residence duration in designated rooms and sending an email notification about any abnormalities of the patient's behavior. For example, (e.g. staying in the restroom for more than an hour).

4 Conclusions

Alzheimer's disease is not just a burden to the patients but also to their family and care givers, Alzheimer's patients need special care twenty-four hours a day. Thus, an indoor localization system comes to the advantage of Alzheimer's patients in ensuring their safety and to advantage of their care taker in convenience. This paper demonstrated that an RFID-based indoor localization system is highly appropriate for guaranteeing the safety of Alzheimer's patients without invading their privacy. Furthermore, the system showed promising results and could easily implement and replicated and doesn't require high level maintenance. Limitation due to body shadowing could be avoided in the future using custom made RFID tags.

Acknowledgment. The authors would like to thank King Fahd University for the support of this project.

References

1. Ranjan, J., Yao, Y., Whitehouse, K.: An RF doormat for tracking people's room locations. In: Proceedings of the 2013 ACM International Joint Conference on Pervasive and Ubiquitous Computing, pp. 797–800. ACM (2013)
2. Saab, S.S., Nakad, Z.S.: A standalone RFID indoor positioning system using passive tags. IEEE Trans. Ind. Electron. **58**, 1961–1970 (2011)
3. Berz, E.L., Tesch, D.A., Hessel, F.P.: RFID indoor localization based on support vector regression and k-means. In: 2015 IEEE 24th International Symposium on Industrial Electronics (ISIE), pp. 1418–1423. IEEE (2015)
4. Kulkarni, A., Sathe, S.: Healthcare applications of the internet of things: a review. Int. J. Comput. Sci. Inf. Technol. **5**, 6229–6232 (2014)
5. Siddagangaiah, S.: A novel approach to IoT based plant health monitoring system (2016)
6. Wang, C., Daneshmand, M., Dohler, M., Mao, X., Hu, R.Q., Wang, H.: Guest editorial-special issue on internet of things (IoT): architecture, protocols and services. IEEE Sensors J. **13**, 3505–3510 (2013)

Automated Recognition and Difficulty Assessment of Boulder Routes

André Ebert(✉) , Kyrill Schmid, Chadly Marouane,
and Claudia Linnhoff-Popien

Institute for Computer Science Mobile and Distributed Systems Group,
Ludwig-Maximilians-University, Oettingenstrasse 67, 80538 Munich, Germany
{andre.ebert,kyrill.schmid,chadly.marouane,linnhoff}@ifi.lmu.de

Abstract. Due to fast distribution of powerful, portable processing
devices and wearables, the development of learning-based IoT-applications
for athletic or medical usage is accelerated. But besides the offering of quantitative features, such as counting repetitions or distances, there are only
a few systems which provide qualitative services, e.g., detecting malposi-
tions to avoid injuries or to optimize training success.

Therefore we present a novel, holistic, and sensor-based approach for
qualitative analysis of asynchronous, non-recurrent human motion. Furthermore, we deploy it to automatically assess the difficulty level of boulder routes on basis of climbing movements. Within a comprehensive study
encompassing 153 ascents of 18 climbers, we extract and examine features
such as strength, endurance, and control and achieve a successful classification rate of difficulty levels of more than 98%.

Keywords: Machine learning · Activity recognition and assessment
Climbing and bouldering

1 Introduction

Applications targeting usage within the athletic context and based on smartphones as well as on wearables are ubiquitous by now. Commonly, they provide
customized workout plans or count quantitative qualities, while the provision of
qualitative feedback exists only sparsely. Therefore, we developed a procedure
for qualitative analysis of climbing motion in order to automatically assess the
difficulty of boulder routes. In that context, the term boulder route comprises
relatively short climbing routes of significantly higher difficulty (compared to
normal climbing routes). Due to their commonly low height, they are climbed
without safety equipment. Because of the varying and merging complexities of
boulder routes as well as the strong dependence on a climber's individual skills,
an impartial assessment of a route's level of difficulty is a tough task. In the best
case, consequences of an incorrect assessment may be the frustration of a climber
or minor injuries due to unfamiliar moves or physical overload. But in the worst
case, severe accidents and fatal injuries may occur (e.g., due to a climber's lack of

© ICST Institute for Computer Sciences, Social Informatics and Telecommunications Engineering 2018
M. U. Ahmed et al. (Eds.): HealthyIoT 2017, LNICST 225, pp. 62–68, 2018.
https://doi.org/10.1007/978-3-319-76213-5_9

skills, wrong appraisal, or hubris) and lead to complex, dangerous, and expensive rescue expeditions.

In order to solve such issues, we developed a distributed sensor system capable of holistic capturing and analysis of recurrent human motion in real-time [1,2]. Now, we extend the underlying concepts and develop a novel procedure for qualitative motion assessment relying on asynchronous, non-recurrent, and multi-dimensional timeseries (see Sect. 3). In order evaluate its capabilities we conducted a study encompassing climbing data of 18 participants for 153 ascents on different boulder routes which are labeled with difficulty levels of the Fontainebleau technical grades scale (see Sect. 4). During analysis we prove that our approach is capable of assessing difficulty levels of boulder routes with a success rate of more than 98%. Finally, Sect. 5 sums up our findings, discusses open issues and provides an outlook onto future research.

2   Related Work

In the following, we present existing work dealing with human activity recognition as well as the analysis of climbing techniques and climbing style. Pansiot et al. show that it is possible to distinguish different climbing styles by extracting features which reflect a climber's fluidity, speed, endurance, and strength-to-weight ratio out of an ear-worn accelerometer [6]. Ladha et al. present ClimbAX, a system which also tries to assess a climber's skills by utilizing similar features extracted from two hand-worn sensors [5]. Both approaches provide interesting input concerning qualitative feature engineering for climbing activities. Kosmalla et al. introduced a concept for automated recognition of climbing routes and presents state-of-art results for that use-case [4]. Still, this approach is not capable of a more generic classification which is necessary to determine a routes level of difficulty in an automated, generic, and precise way. In [2] we present a distributed sensor system called SensX, which allows to capture the whole human body's acceleration and rotation information among other data (i.e., lighting, temperature, barometric pressure, etc.). In [1] we utilize this system as a basis for qualitatively assessing complex and recurrent human motion and demonstrate its capabilities for the use-case of body weight exercises. Thereby, we present state-of-the-art results with a successful classification rate of 99.3% for qualitative assessment and 100% for sheer activity recognition. Though this concept is not suitable for processing asynchronous, non-recurrent motion information, it still functions as a basis for our concept, which is introduced in the following.

3   A Concept for Automated Assessment of Boulder Routes

In contrast to the assessment of recurrent human motion as proposed in [2] climbing activities may not be described by features like similarity, periodicity, or runtime. One reason for the difficulty of using temporal features is that different boulder and climbing routes are of significantly varying lengths and consistencies. Together with skill-dependent ascent times, that makes it hard to find generalizable, time-dependent features for a whole climbing activity. The lack of periodicity results in the fact, that comparison to qualitatively labeled patterns is also not feasible, e.g., a pushup of good quality vs. one of bad quality. To overcome those issues, we use some assumptions based on climbing theory: an increased level of route difficulty is indicated by inaccurate gripping and increased use of strength during transition periods, while a trembling of the climber's limbs occurs more often within rest periods because of exhaustion and imperfect control. The core skills *control, stability, speed,* and *economical use of strength* are harder to achieve for difficult routes and therefore seem suitable as a theoretical basis for feature engineering [3,5,6].

3.1 Tracking Human Motion Information

In order to track rotation, acceleration, and temporal information occurring while climbing, we applied the SensX sensor architecture mentioned in Sect. 2 as a technical basis. It allows tracking of the human body's limbs and provides an integrated device for realtime processing of incoming sensor data. The four external MBientLab sensor platforms (right arm, left arm, right leg, left leg) provide sample rates of roughly 40 Hz while the processing unit (chest) provides 50 Hz for acceleration and 100 Hz for rotation data. All devices are connected by Bluetooth Low Energy (BLE) and are synchronized by the processing unit. Output of the SensX system are 30 individual sensor data streams: acceleration (X-, Y-, and Z-axis) and rotation (X-, Y-, Z-axis) for 4 external sensor platforms plus the processing unit.

3.2 Preprocessing and Feature Engineering

Subsequently, we describe our advance towards the extraction of an expressive feature set. First, the actual climbing activity is identified and segmented into transition and rest periods (see Sect. 3 and Fig. 1a). Afterwards, we extract our features needed later on for supervised learning.

Segmentation. Generally, a climbing activity takes place in between a temporal interval Δt and has a start time t_s as well as an end time t_e. For further analysis, this interval needs to be distinguished from interfering activities first, e.g., walking or standing. Therefore, an extended approach of [5] respecting the climber's hands positions for activity recognition is utilized: Fig. 1a depicts the acceleration of the right hand including t_{sr} and t_{er}. Within our sensor setup, the hand's acceleration along the Y-axis indicates, whether the climber's arm is currently oriented upwards or downwards.

Using that assumption, we sequentially process the acceleration information of both hands in an overlapping sliding window of 750 ms length. If the mean acceleration in a frame is greater than zero, the arm points upwards and a

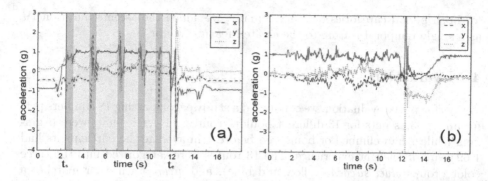

Fig. 1. (a) Acceleration of the right hand during a boulder session with rest (green) and transition periods (grey), (b) shows the chest sensors acceleration. (Color figure online)

describing flag f is set `true`. If both arms point upwards for multiple frames, the climbing activity has started and t_s is marked by the beginning of the first frames where f_r and f_l are `true`. The climbing activity ends as soon as both hands are pointing downwards for multiple frames, whereby t_e is indicated by the beginning of the first frames where f_r and f_l are `false`. In order to prepare for the actual feature extraction, the climbing activity now becomes segmented into rest and transition periods. The sum of the acceleration's standard deviations (X, Y, Z) indicates the released energy potential for each window frame: $S = S_x + S_y + S_z$. If S is greater than an empirically determined threshold, the frame belongs to a transition period, else it indicates a rest period.

Feature Extraction. Based on the core skills mentioned in Sect. 3, we extracted 163 features for each boulder route out of the before segmented rest and transition periods. Each external platform, is described by $2 * 9 * 2 = 36$ features (9 transition period features and 9 rest period features for acceleration and rotation, respectively). Broken down to each period category we use (1) the average means of all axis m_x, m_y, and m_z, (2) their standard deviations s_x, s_y, s_z, (3) the maximum value of the individual sums of all standard deviations of all existing periods within a category s_{smax}, (4) their average mean s_{smean} and (5) the standard deviation of all sums of standard deviations s_{sstd}. E.g., in case of transition periods, consistent values for (1) and (2) imply a stable *control* and *stability*, while (3), (4), and (5) give hints onto the amount of expended energy and therefore strength. In case of rest periods, a higher value implies a lack of control and stability. As depicted in Fig. 1a, the information provided by the processing unit's sensors is much less distinct than that of the external sensor devices (see Fig. 1b). This makes it hard to categorize it into transition and rest periods. Reason for that is the fact that during climbing the limbs are much more in motion than the chest. Therefore, we extracted only 18 features for both period categories together. Finally, we added the ascents duration Δt as a single temporal feature to the created feature vector.

4 Evaluation

For performance evaluation, we conducted a study encompassing 18 climbers performing 153 ascents for 13 different boulder routes. 11 participants were beginners while 7 had climbed or bouldered before – in average the participants had 1.69 years of relevant experience. The 13 routes were categorized into the three color groups *blue*, *sweden* (yellow and blue), and *green*. Each color matches a difficulty range of Fontainebleau technical grades, the most widely used grading system for boulder routes in Europe. According to that, blue is mapped to the grades 1a-2c, sweden encompasses 3a-4b and green matches 4b-5c. In order to enable as much participants as possible to complete the whole study, the tracked routes were of comparably low difficulty.

4.1 Automated Identification of Difficulty Levels

During evaluation, we utilized different supervised machine learning algorithms which are common in related work as well as AutoWeka for automated hyper parameter optimization (HPO). Preceding experiences during the analysis of recurrent timeseries made us assume initially that a sensor setup which covers all limbs as well as an athlete's chest is perfect analyzing athletic movements. But as depicted in Fig. 1c, the chest sensor provides only vague information for climbing activities (e.g., compared to the hand sensor, see Fig. 1a). Hence, we developed a more fine-grained evaluation approach and examined different sensor configurations as well as their influence onto the classification results, as shown in Table 1. As indicated before, the inclusion of the chest sensor's features never improves the results significantly (see Random Forest (RF), Support Vector Machine (SVM)) while in other cases the results are even better if the chest features are not observed at all (see C4.5, Naive Bayes (NB), HPO). In general, the chest sensor's features achieve comparably low success rates if examined isolated. The best results are achieved by using only the limb's features and

Table 1. Classification results for different classifiers and sensor configurations (all sensors, hands only, legs only, chest only, limbs only) and the average training time.

Classifier	All	Top	Bottom	Chest	Limbs	Duration (avg.)
Random Forest	79.74%	74.51%	71.24%	64.71%	79.01%	104 ms
C4.5	67.32%	57.52%	58.82%	56.73%	68.63%	20 ms
Support Vector	86.93%	74.51%	85.0%	75.82%	86.27%	40 ms
Naive Bayes	71.24%	66.67%	62.09%	49.02%	75.82%	8 ms
HPO	89.54%	79.74%	82.34%	60.78%	98.04%	327 ms

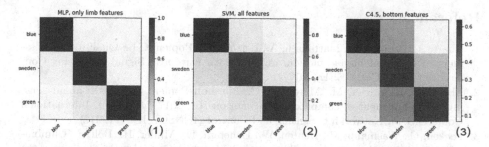

Fig. 2. Confusion matrices for classification results: (1) MLP and only limb features; (2) SVM and all features; (3) C4.5 and only bottom features. (Color figure online)

building our model with an hyper parameter optimized Multilayer Perceptron (MLP), a neural network which has a nonlinear activation function and utilizes backpropagation for training purposes. Hence, we are able to classify the difficulty level of different routes with a success rate of 98.04%. Figure 2 shows the distribution of classified instances for different setups and classifiers within confusion matrices. Especially in (3) it is strongly apparent, that wrongly classified instances are mostly assigned to a neighboring level of difficulty. This illustrates that a color always contains a range of difficulty grades and that neighboring colors may also encompass intersecting grades.

5   Conclusion

Within this paper, we presented a novel approach for analyzing asynchronous and non-recurrent human motion. Therefore, we first track climbing motion with the SensX sensor system, then we detect and segment climbing activities from interfering activities and develop an expressive feature set which is capable of describing non-recurrent and asynchronous human motion, i.e., climbing, in a qualitative way. To validate our approach and to demonstrate its capabilities, we conduct a comprehensive study and classify different difficulty levels of boulder routes with a success rate of more than 98%.

But despite these promising results, we are also aware of still unsolved challenges. E.g., a more fine grained classification concept could solve issues with incorrect assignments of instances to neighboring difficulty levels. Moreover, we currently regard only routes of easy and intermediate difficulty while characteristics of tough routes such as strongly overhanging rocks and tiny grips are not depicted within our feature set. These issues as well as others are subject of ongoing research.

References

1. Ebert, A., Beck, M.T., Mattausch, A., Belzner, L., Popien, C.L.: Qualitative assessment of recurrent human motion. In: 2017 25th European Signal Processing Conference (EUSIPCO). IEEE (2017)
2. Ebert, A., Kiermeier, M., Marouane, C., Linnhoff-Popien, C.: SensX: about sensing and assessment of complex human motion. In: 2017 14th IEEE International Conference on Networking, Sensing and Control (ICNSC). IEEE (2017)
3. Feeken, C., Wasmann, M., Heuten, W., Ennenga, D., Müller, H., Boll, S.: ClimbingAssist: direct vibro-tactile feedback on climbing technique. In: Proceedings of the 2016 ACM International Joint Conference on Pervasive and Ubiquitous Computing: Adjunct, pp. 57–60. ACM (2016)
4. Kosmalla, F., Daiber, F., Krüger, A.: ClimbSense: automatic climbing route recognition using wrist-worn inertia measurement units. In: Proceedings of the 33rd Annual ACM Conference on Human Factors in Computing Systems. ACM (2015)
5. Ladha, C., Hammerla, N.Y., Olivier, P., Plötz, T.: ClimbAX: skill assessment for climbing enthusiasts. In: Proceedings of the 2013 ACM International Joint Conference on Pervasive and Ubiquitous Computing, pp. 235–244. ACM (2013)
6. Pansiot, J., King, R.C., McIlwraith, D.G., Lo, B.P., Yang, G.Z.: ClimBSN: climber performance monitoring with BSN. In: 5th International Summer School and Symposium on Medical Devices and Biosensors, 2008. ISSS-MDBS 2008, pp. 33–36. IEEE (2008)

e-PWV: A Web Application for Assessing Online Carotid-Femoral Pulse Wave Velocity

Mathieu Collette[1,2](✉), Naoures Hassine[1], Carlo Palombo[3], and Georges Leftheriotis[4,5]

[1] Groupe ESAIP, 18 rue du 8 Mai 1945,
BP 80022, 49192 Saint Barthélemy d'Anjou, France
collettemathieu@noolib.com
[2] Laboratoire Angevin de Recherche en Ingènierie des Systémes (LARIS),
Université d'Angers, 62 Avenue Notre Dame du Lac, 49000 Angers, France
[3] Department of Surgical, Medical, Molecular Pathology and Critical Care Medicine,
University of Pisa, Via Savi 10, 56126 Pisa, Italy
[4] Université de Nice, LP2M-CNRS-UNS UMR 7370,
Faculté de Médecine, 28, Avenue de Valombrose, 06107 Nice, France
[5] CHU de Nice, Unité d'Explorations Fonctionnelles Vasculaires,
30 voie romaine, 06000 Nice, France

Abstract. This article presents e-PWV, a web application for the determination of Pulse Wave Velocity (PWV) running on a web platform called NooLib. e-PWV has been applied on signals recorded by an ultrasound system (PWV_{et}, Aloka, Japan) and representing the arterial diameter changes in carotid and femoral sites. PWV_{et} measurements were compared to PWV recorded by a tonometric technique (PWV_{pp}, PulsePen, Italy). The study was conducted on 120 patients. We found an excellent correlation of r = 0.95 between PWV_{et} et PWV_{pp} ($P < 0.0001$; 95% confidence interval of 0.91–0.96; $PWV_{et} = 0.88 \times PWV_{pp} + 0.57$). We observed a small offset of $-0.33 \, \mathrm{ms}^{-1}$ on the Bland-Altman plot with a limit of agreement from -2.21 to $1.54 \, \mathrm{ms}^{-1}$. Our results suggest that e-PWV application can produce online a reliable marker of the regional aortic stiffness using an echotracking system.

Keywords: Arterial stiffness · Echo-tracking · Ultrasound · Web

1 Introduction

Nowadays, arterial stiffness plays a major role in the development of cardiovascular diseases [1]. Carotid-femoral Pulse Wave Velocity (PWV) represents the most established index of regional aortic stiffness and numerous techniques

The authors would like to thank all ESAIP students who have contributed to the development of the NooLib platform, the Clinical Pathophysiology Laboratory of the University of Pisa and the Clinical Research Center of Angers (France).

© ICST Institute for Computer Sciences, Social Informatics and Telecommunications Engineering 2018
M. U. Ahmed et al. (Eds.): HealthyIoT 2017, LNICST 225, pp. 69–74, 2018.
https://doi.org/10.1007/978-3-319-76213-5_10

allow its determination non-invasively [2]. These techniques rely generally on the recording of one or several arterial hemodynamic parameters (pressure, velocity or diameter) and embed a software for the automatic computing of pulse wave velocity based on a foot-to-foot method [3].

We present, here, a web application, called e-PWV, allowing the online assessment of the pulse wave velocity between two arterial sites. The application runs on a homemade web platform, called NooLib. NooLib can host algorithms coming from scientific research and transform them in an easy to use application. NooLib ensures the data security and intellectual property of algorithms since all applications run on the server side in a Linux container.

In practice, e-PWV needs one signal per arterial site representing an arterial hemodynamic parameter as a function of time and synchronized with the electrocardiogram (ECG) signal. Thereafter, the application applies an intersecting tangent algorithm in order to detect, for each site, the foot of the waveform. The transit time Δt between the two sites is computed as the time delay between the feet of the waveforms and the velocity is deduced as the ratio between the distance d and Δt where d represents the distance between the two anatomical sites.

In this article, e-PWV has been developed because no algorithm is currently embedded in ultrasound systems for the determination of carotid-femoral PWV. Actually, ultrasound systems (B-mode) that can implement echo-tracking technology (ET) allow visualization of the blood vessels. The recording of local diameter changes in peripheral arteries (namely carotid or femoral arteries) is feasible. Then, the carotid and femoral diameter waveforms can be saved separately in a text file and the transit time between the two sites can be computed from a foot-to-foot method.

A bicentric study was conducted with the hospital of Angers (France) and the university of Pisa (Italy) in order to validate this approach. The study was developed to assess the accuracy and repeatability of carotid-femoral PWV measurements using the e-PWV application as compared to the reference tonometric technique [4].

2   Materials and Methods

2.1   The NooLib Platform

The NooLib platform (www.noolib.com) has two goals:

1. For non-developers: offer them the opportunity to use algorithms without skills in programming languages.
2. For developers: have a better interaction with the users and the applications on the platform.

NooLib therefore represents a collaborative platform where research can be shared and compared through the use of applications online.

Technically, NooLib is a web platform, currently in beta, which enables researchers to deposit algorithms written in Java/Python/Javascript/PHP or

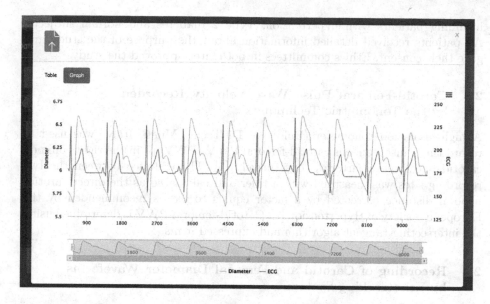

Fig. 1. The data manager on the NooLib platform. We can see two signals coming from echotracking technology representing the arterial diameter changes and the ECG signal. The x-axis represents time in second and the y-axis is graduated according to data loaded (in mm for the arterial diameter changes and arbitrary unit for the ECG signal). Before injecting data into an application, we can select an appropriate interval and save it.

Matlab and transform them into an application with an user-friendly interface. The kernel of the platform relies on an operating-system-level virtualization method for running multiple isolated Linux systems on a control host using a single Linux kernel. The Linux kernel provides a control group functionality that allows limitation and prioritization of resources (CPU, memory, block I/O, network, etc.). Then, NooLib enables each algorithm to be run on the server side in an isolated environment maintaining a high degree of security and ensures intellectual property rights for users.

A data manger is present on the platform in order to offer the opportunity for users to upload their data before being used in an application online. This allows applications to avoid a pre-control of data before running and for users to select and apply pre-processing on data before injecting them into an application (see Fig. 1). Currently, the data manager allows uploading files in csv, txt or edf format and images in jpg, jpg2000, png or Dicom format.

2.2 Population Studied

A total of 120 patients (69 men) between 18 and 81 years of age (mean age: 43 ± 18 years) were enrolled to the study. The population was initially referred for vascular screening for atherosclerosis, metabolic disease or inherited diseases including patients with hypertension, Type 2 diabetes and normal subjects. All patients received detailed information about the purpose of the study and gave their consent. Ethics committees in both sites approved the study.

2.3 Carotid-Femoral Pulse Wave Velocity Recorded by the Tonometric Technique

A high-resolution tonometer (Pulsepen, DiaTecne, Milan, Italy) was used to record the transcutaneous carotid-femoral PWV (PWVpp) in the right common carotid and femoral arteries consecutively [5]. The distance between the two recording sites was measured with a ruler and calculated as the direct carotid-femoral distance corrected by a factor equals to 0.8 as recommended by the European Society of Hypertension [3]. Carotid-femoral PWV is determined using the intersecting tangent algorithm and expressed in ms^{-1}.

2.4 Recording of Carotid and Femoral Diameter Waveforms by Echotracking System

The ECG signal, the carotid diameter waveform and the femoral diameter waveform were obtained by a high-resolution ET ultrasound system (US) coupled to a standard B-mode imaging (Alpha 10, Aloka, Japan). To track the displacement of arterial walls during cardiac cycle, wall-tracking calipers were set to the intima-media interface of the near and far arterial wall, and wall movements were followed automatically by the system with high spatial and temporal resolution. The carotid and femoral diameter changes were exported in text format for an importation in NooLib.

2.5 Carotid-Femoral Pulse Wave Velocity Using e-PWV Application

e-PWV has been written in Python 3. The application allows a sample rate parameter which can be adjusted in NooLib before running the application. It represents the sample rate of signals inputted into the application. A low-pass filter with a cutoff frequency at 40 Hz is applied on each signals received in order to improve the signal to noise ratio. A first algorithm detects each R-peaks of ECG signal and each cardiac cycle is isolated for the carotid and the femoral arteries. Then, the carotid and femoral distension waveforms were averaged over ten cardiac cycles. In the case where less than ten cardiac cycles are detected, e-PWV performs an average over the total of cardiac cycles detected. A second algorithm, based on an intersecting tangent method, was applied to the mean curves in order to detect the feet of the carotid and femoral waveforms. The calculation of PWV_{et} was established as the ratio between the distance of the two sites (carotid and femoral arterial sites) and the time delay evaluated between the feet of the waveforms. The distance between the two sites was the same as used for the PWV_{pp} value using the tonometric technique in order to prevent bias between both techniques.

2.6 Comparison of PWV_{pp} and PWV_{et}

Two consecutive ET and tonometric measurements were carried out by experienced operators (C. Palombo and G. Leftheriotis). The mean of the 2 measurements was retained for our analysis. ET and tonometric examinations were made in random order. The systolic and diastolic brachial arterial blood pressures were collected by an automatic sphygmomanometer (Welch-Allyn, NY, USA) with an appropriate cuff size.

2.7 Statistical Analysis

All statistical analyses were performed with the Prism software (GraphPad, La Jolla, CA, version 5.0). Agreement between PWV_{pp} and PWV_{et} variables was assessed using a Student's paired t-tests and Bland-Altman plots. The relationship among PWV_{pp} and PWV_{et} was evaluated by linear regression. Repeatability of PWV_{pp} and PWV_{et} measurements were estimated by calculating a within-subject coefficient of variation for repeated measurements and Bland-Altman plots. For all statistics, a P value of <0.05 was considered statistically significant.

3 Results

The biometric and hemodynamic characteristics of the patients are presented in Table 1. PWVpp and PWVet measurements showed respectively a good signal-to-noise ratio of 91% and 94% of the recordings. It was only when wave foot detection was feasible that PWV_{pp} and PWV_{et} were taken into account in the statistical analysis.

No significant difference was observed between the mean PWV_{pp} (7.40 ± 2.85 ms^{-1}) and the mean PWV_{et} (7.06 ± 2.61 ms^{-1}). We found a significant Pearson correlation coefficient of $r = 0.94$ between the 2 variables ($P < 0.0001$; 95% confidence interval 0.91–0.96; $PWV_{et} = 0.88 \times PWV_{pp} + 0.57$). The Bland-Altman plot showed a small offset of -0.33 ms^{-1} with a limit of agreement from -2.21 to 1.54 ms^{-1} between the 2 variables.

Table 1. Main clinical characteristics of patients. Results are displayed as Mean±SD and Mann-Whitney t-test: *$P < 0.05$ vs overall population **$P < 0.01$ vs overall population ***$P < 0.001$ vs overall population

Parameter	Overall (n = 120)	Pisa (n = 80)	Angers (n = 40)
Age	43 ± 18	38 ± 18*	52 ± 15**
Systolic blood pressure (mmHg)	119 ± 14	118 ± 14	121 ± 13
Diastolic blood pressure (mmHg)	72 ± 10	71 ± 10	75 ± 10
PWV_{pp} (m/s)	7.40 ± 2.85	6.05 ± 1.70**	10.04 ± 2.80***
PWV_{et} (m/s)	7.06 ± 2.61	5.76 ± 1.50***	9.52 ± 2.51***

For all participants, we observed a small coefficient of variation of 5.8% and 8.5% between two consecutive carotid-femoral PWV_{et} and PWV_{pp} respectively, without significant differences in the within-subject repeatability. Finally, comparing two successive PWV_{pp} measurements, the Bland-Altman plot showed a small offset of $-0.08\,\text{ms}^{-1}$ with a limit of agreement from -2.11 to $1.95\,\text{ms}^{-1}$. The same analysis showed a systematic offset of $0.14\,\text{ms}^{-1}$ with a limit of agreement from -1.71 to $2.00\,\text{ms}^{-1}$ for two successive PWV_{et} measurements.

4   Conclusion

The accuracy of the ET technique in the assessment of the carotid-femoral PWV using e-PWV application was demonstrated in this study showing an excellent correlation with the tonometric technique. The Bland and Altman analysis also revealed a small offset between both techniques and the repeatability between the two techniques showed no significant difference. The results may indicate that tonometric techniques and ultrasound system could be interchangeable. This leads to the conclusion that e-PWV application on NooLib can compute online a reliable marker of the carotid-femoral PWV using an echo-tracking system. Thereafter, e-PWV could be validated for other technologies recording an hemodynamic parameter of the artery coupled to an ECG signal. For example, tonometric signals could also be extracted for an analysis online of the aortic stiffness using the e-PWV application.

References

1. Simon, A.C., Levenson, J., Bouthier, J., Safar, M.E., Avolio, A.P.: Evidence of early degenerative changes in large arteries in human essential hypertension. Hypertension 7, 675–680 (1985)
2. Willum, H.T., Staessen, J., Torp-Pedersen, C., Rasmussen, S., Thijs, L., Ibsen, H., Jeppesen, J.: Prognostic value of aortic pulse wave velocity as index of arterial stiffness in the general population. Circulation 113, 664–670 (2006)
3. Van Bortel, L.M., Laurent, S., Boutouyrie, P., Chowienczyk, P., Cruickshank, J.K., De Backer, T., Filipovsky, J., Huybrechts, S., Mattace-Raso, F.U., Protogerou, A.D., Schillaci, G., Segers, P., Vermeersch, S., Weber, T.: Expert consensus document on the measurement of aortic stiffness in daily practice using carotid-femoral pulse wave velocity. J. Hypertens. 30, 445–448 (2012)
4. Agnoletti, D., Millasseau, S.C., Topouchian, J., Zhang, Y., Safar, M.E., Blacher, J.: Pulse wave analysis with two tonometric devices: a comparison study. Physiol. Meas. 35, 1837 (2014)
5. Salvi, P., Lio, G., Labat, C., Ricci, E., Pannier, B., Benetos, A.: Validation of a new non-invasive portable tonometer for determining arterial pressure wave and pulse wave velocity: the PulsePen device. J. Hypertens. 22, 2285–2293 (2004)

Automatic Autism Spectrum Disorder Detection Thanks to Eye-Tracking and Neural Network-Based Approach

Romuald Carette[1]([✉]), Federica Cilia[2], Gilles Dequen[1], Jerome Bosche[1], Jean-Luc Guerin[1], and Luc Vandromme[2]

[1] Laboratoire Modélisation, Information et Systèmes,
Université de Picardie Jules Verne, Amiens, Picardie, France
{romuald.carette,gilles.dequen,jerome.bosche,
jean-luc.guerin}@u-picardie.fr
[2] Centre de Recherche en Psychologie: Cognition, Psychisme et Organisations,
Université de Picardie Jules Verne, Amiens, Picardie, France
{federica.cilia,luc.vandromme}@u-picardie.fr

Abstract. Autism spectrum disorder (ASD) is a neurodevelopmental disorder quite wide and its numerous variations render diagnosis hard. Some works have proven that children suffering from autism have trouble keeping their attention and tend to have a less focused sight. On top of that, eye-tracking systems enable the recording of precise eye focus on a screen. This paper deals with automatic detection of autism spectrum disorder thanks to eye-tracked data and an original Machine Learning approach. Focusing on data that describes the saccades of the patient's sight, we distinguish, out of our six test patients, young autistic individuals from those with no problems in 83% (five) of tested patients, with a results confidence up to 95%.

Keywords: Neural network · Long Short-Term Memory (LSTM)
Data processing · Eye-tracking · Autism spectrum disorder · eHealth

1 Introduction

The notion of autism spectrum disorder implies different profiles in this disorder, shared by 1% of the world's population. Even though it is possible to detect at an early age, the methods used for this detection are, to date, mainly manual like parents interview or observations. As a decision support, a system called *eye-tracker* allows the reading of patients sight on a screen. It displays a set of information including the pixel each eye is aiming at, the gaze state, the position of patient's eyes, the pupil size and position, etc. As raw data, the system considers a set of three states: fixation, saccade and blink. While "fixation" and "saccade" represent sequential data with eye-focus staying into an area

The work presented in this paper is supported by Evolucare Technologies grant.

© ICST Institute for Computer Sciences, Social Informatics and Telecommunications Engineering 2018
M. U. Ahmed et al. (Eds.): HealthyIoT 2017, LNICST 225, pp. 75–81, 2018.
https://doi.org/10.1007/978-3-319-76213-5_11

for the first, continuously moving for the latter, "blink" is quite different [1]. This state indicates the lost track of the eye, without knowing whether the patient actually blinked or just turned his/her head. It has been found that the dispersion of the patient's eye focus helps to indicate whether he/she is affected by an autism spectrum disorder. Research points towards this idea to find applicable solutions in diagnosis. These types of solutions remain manual, requiring data reading and expertise to be sure of a patient's situation. We propose an automatic approach based on LSTM neural networks and focusing on the saccade part of the readings. Our resulting solution ends up validating the state of 83% of the patients. Section 2 focuses on the autism spectrum disorder and the eye-tracker system. Section 3 provides a description of Neural Networks. In Sect. 4, we describe our approach and Sect. 5 provides some experimental results. We finally conclude and provide some future works in Sect. 6.

2   Autism Spectrum Disorder and Eye-Tracker System

In this section, we will state what autism spectrum disorder is, present the complexity of its diagnosis, and the eye-tracker system considered in our situation.

2.1   Autism Spectrum Disorder

Autism spectrum disorders are expressed notably through limited capacities for communication and social interaction, linked to difficulty for making eye contact with others. These difficulties can be demonstrated, for example, by analyzing family films, which highlight an abnormal visual behavior towards others, in persons with autism spectrum disorders [2], as well as a preference for non social stimuli over social stimuli such as faces [3]. This preference may be explained by a specific deficit in processing faces [4], leading to recognition disorders [5]. However, deficits at a lower level, such as perceptive and/or attentional ones [6] put a question mark over the indispensable prerequisites in building these processing capacities in the child with autism spectrum disorders. In this regard, systematic studies of visual activity in persons with autism spectrum disorder, carried out using recordings of visual activity (eye-tracking), regularly highlight unadapted visual exploration strategies [7]. Nonetheless, heterogeneous or even contradictory results do not allow any conclusions to be reached concerning the quality of visual exploration of faces by persons with autism spectrum disorders. While specific patterns of visual activity depending on groups are sometimes demonstrated, they are not systematically replicated: the results could be dependent on the age of the participants, on the severity of their disorder and/or on their cognitive ability, but also on the type of stimuli used (static versus dynamic) or on the task required (free exploration, recognizing faces or emotional expressions, etc.) For a review, see Falck-Ytter and von Hofsten [8]. Results of studies using dynamic social stimuli come out for the most part in favor of atypical visual exploration of participants with autism spectrum disorders compared to control participants, notably with a diminution in eye fixation time [9].

2.2   Eye-Tracker System

Oculometry (eye-tracking or gaze-tracking) combines a group of techniques allowing eye movements to be recorded. Combined with pupillometry, these techniques are currently used in a variety of fields such as psychology and psycholinguistics, as well as experiencing a considerable momentum in the field of neurosciences and physiology. In the field of autism, these non-invasive techniques are currently used to improve diagnosis and therapeutic strategies through a better understanding of the physiopathological and psychological mechanisms which underlay the observed symptoms. This technique allows the ocular activity of an individual to be analyzed, demonstrating where his eyes are fixing, and thus revealing what he is and what he is not looking at. It enriches the more traditional methods of observation by allowing assessment of what a person is looking at while carrying out a cognitive and/or relational activity. It is a tool among others allowing the assessment and understanding of human activity as well as the analysis of a percept.

Within this study, visual activity has been recorded with a sampling frequency of 60 Hz using the SMI RED250mobile IView XTM RED device.

3   About Neural Networks

Neural Networks are state-of-the-art tools from the Artificial Intelligence field. Mimicking the functioning of the human brain, it takes given data as input and results in the form needed by its creator as output, transitioning the information though nodes and weighted connections (like brain cells and synapses). After a step of training (or learning), the network is ready to interpret any set of additional data to give the expected answer. That answer can be of many forms: a prediction, a classification or just a correlated value.

Many different implementations of Neural Networks exist. From Artificial Neural Network (ANN, Fig. 1a), Recurrent Neural Networks (RNNs, Fig. 1b) have been created. Due to RNNs limitations, LSTMs have been proposed. More robust than their past implementation, LSTMs are also harder to train [10]. A

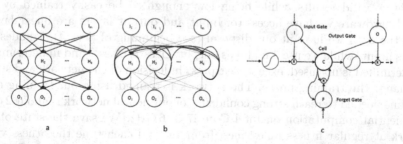

Fig. 1. (a) A ANN with m input nodes, n output nodes and a single hidden layer of k nodes ; (b) Same as (a), but as a RNN, recurrent connections are bold ; (c) A LSTM node, the inputs are dotted, the output is long-dotted

LSTM follows the implementation of a classic RNN, except from some specific nodes. Said nodes are now called cells as they are more complex: a cell is preceded and followed by other nodes (fed respectively by an input gate and an output gate), one more node is used as memory eraser (fed by a forget gate). The gates, as well as the entrance of the cell, are all given the same set of data. One single output then gets out of the ensemble. The cell is connected to every gate. In comparison with a classic node, a cell is itself constituted of more connections (see Fig. 1c).

4   Our Approach

The training and test patients are from 8 to 10 years old. We have their data divided between two classes, namely autistic (class 1) and typical (class 2). We studied a total of 17 children from class 1 and 15 from class 2. The first step of work is to capture the data from the patients. To do that, each child is placed in front of a prerecorded video of a joint attention offer, staring a person who performs some actions: showing or speaking about a balloon, which may visible or not. Every child is shown the same order of actions. Each action should lead the child to look at some element of the video. If it is visible, the child should focus on it, else, he/she may search on the screen for the element. All tracking information are recorded by an eye-tracking system. The data we choose to focus on is the saccadic movement of the eye. This includes the amplitude, the acceleration (average and maximum), the deceleration (maximum), the velocity (average and maximum), the rate of maximum velocity for a given saccade and the duration of the saccade. Gathered data is used anonymously for privacy reasons. Instead we use a color as name. To be easily usable in our specific LSTM network, data is normalized so that each value is included in [0,1]. Data is divided between two sets, training and testing data (resp. about 75% and 25%). Test data consists in 4 patients from class 1 and 3 patients from class 2. We implement our solution within Pybrain module[1] framework, using the LSTM Layers it provides. Due to the sequenced data we use, we work with a network made of LSTM hidden layers. The hidden layers consists of 2 LSTM layers composed of 20 nodes each. These nodes amounts are high enough to provide us valid results, while being low enough to be easily trained by the limited hardware we have access to. Input and output layers are linear layers. Given the data we have at our disposal (see beginning of Sect. 4), 7 nodes are used as input, while we use 3 nodes as output: class 1, class 2 and undetermined. Undetermined is not used, except to express indecision of the network and seems to enhance the training phase. The network is trained using our training data set. Time needed to reach strong confidence of our neural network is about 2 days of sequential computation on Intel Core i7 3, 6 GHz. We save the state of the network at regular fitness milestones, from 1.0 and each time the fitness value decreases by 0.001 after that. A state includes the fitness milestone reached, the evaluations for the test data set, the validation rate, the average certainty of the

---

[1] http://pybrain.org/ version 0.3.

evaluations and the current values of the weights of the network (see 5 for said values, excepting weights). We end the training of the network at a 0.004 fitness value. Following the training on the initial patients data, additional patients are used for confirmation of the training. The same information is saved.

5   Experimental Results

We extract the network states with a fitness value from 0.008 to 0.004. We apply this network state to six additional patients to check its validity. Patients are classified into different learned classes: while DarkBlue/DarkCyan/CyanTRIS are TS (diagnosed autism), Cyan/CyanBIS/DarkRed are TC (typical children with the same chronological age without autistic history). The calculation of the TC or TS probabilities are computed as follows: for a given patient, our network returns a value for class 1 (TS), class 2 (TC), class 3 (undefined). Each of these three values are in [0,1]. Then, the probability of class i can be retrieved by dividing the output i by the sum of all outputs. For example, if results are 0.2, 0.55 and 0.05, the patient is recognized as 25% TS, 68.75% TC and 6.25% of pure uncertainty. To make the results more readable, only the highest probability is shown for each case in Table 1. Also, the last column indicates the average confidence on the valid result, thus it is not a mean of the listed confidences. Indeed, on mistakes, the valid result confidence can be very low.

Also, Table 2 shows the confusion matrix of the results from the test data.

We observe that, from fitness values 0.008 to 0.006, 5 of the six patients' diagnosis are confirmed. When the fitness value reaches 0.005, the network suffers from a over-fitting issue. Indeed, we observe that the test data for DarkCyan patient becomes uncertain at 0.005, then gets into the wrong class at 0.004. The confidence then falls to 67%. We notice the highest confidence of the network at over 90% on average, 98% at best (for 0.006 fitness value and 5 over 6 valid

Table 1. Additional patients results

	TS children			TC children			
Fitness	CyanTRIS	DarkBlue	DarkCyan	Cyan	CyanBIS	DarkRed	Avg. Conf.
0.008	TS (88%)	TS (79%)	TS (94%)	TC (70%)	TS (92%)	TC (77%)	67.3%
0.007	TS (88%)	TS (86%)	TS (96%)	TC (73%)	TS (93%)	TC (87%)	66.3%
0.006	TS (89%)	TS (92%)	TS (98%)	TC (78%)	TS (94%)	TC (94%)	65.7%
0.005	TS (92%)	TS (97%)	TS (56%)	TC (79%)	TS (95%)	TC (90%)	60.1%
0.004	TS (95%)	TS (98%)	TC (89%)	TC (81%)	TS (95%)	TC (87%)	54.6%

Table 2. Confusion matrix for network between 0.008 and 0.005 fitness values

	TS Class	TC Class
TS patient	3	0
TC patient	1	2

results), while the mistake result (CyanBis) is strong (94%). On further analysis, we note, in the best case, a sensitivity value at 0.75 and a specificity value at 1.

6   Conclusion and Future Works

We have established that a neural network can distinguish the autism status of young patients thanks to the eye movement of the children. It might help to give a preemptive idea about further analysis to consider for a child who presents signs of this disorder. Such a system could be used with a desktop computer for testing kids at an early age, for example at school. It would be a solution to find more easily ASD suffering children, transmitting relevant data to a professional, including a more in-depth test if necessary. However, the system proposed here is not supposed to replace the work of professionals of the medical field. The help given only consists on an automatic way to focus as fast as possible on the needing children, and maybe point at false diagnoses. Our system works within its current state that has been defined arbitrarily. Still, further work should aim at optimizing the network topology, including the type of nodes used in it and/or the size of layers and their amount. A study on other machine learning solutions should also be conducted, to check the overall efficiency of LSTM-RNNs. Another issue consists in the very low amount of training data, for a neural network approach. Uncertainty and over-fitting might be reduced or removed if more data is gathered for training. Also, we must recall that various rates of autism spectrum disorder exist. Our present solution only gives an idea about the autism status: suffering from it or not. An analogous system might give an early direction about which autistic rate is actually from.

References

1. Cilia, F., Deschamps, L., Vandromme, L.: Investigation of interactive visual patterns during semi-structured joint attention sequences in children with Autism Spectrum Disorder. In: RIPSYDEVE Conference, Louvain-la-neuve (2016)
2. Adrien, J.L., Faure, M., Perrot, A., Hameury, L., Garreau, B., Barthelemy, C., Sauvage, D.: Autism and family home movies: preliminary findings. J. Autism Dev. Disord. 21(1), 43–49 (1991)
3. Maestro, S., Muratori, F., Cesari, A., Pecini, C., Apicella, F., Stern, D.: A view to regressive autism through home movies. is early development really normal? Acta Psychiatrica Scandinavica 113(1), 68–72 (2006)
4. Hobson, R.P., Ouston, J., Lee, A.: What's in a face? the case of autism. Br. J. Psychol. 79(4), 441–453 (1988)
5. Trepagnier, C., Sebrechts, M.M., Peterson, R.: Atypical face gaze in autism. Cyberpsychol. Behav. 5(3), 213–217 (2002)
6. Jemel, B., Mottron, L., Dawson, M.: Impaired face processing in autism: fact or artifact? J. Autism Dev. Disord. 36(1), 91–106 (2006)
7. Pelphrey, K.A., Sasson, N.J., Reznick, J.S., Paul, G., Goldman, B.D., Piven, J.: Visual scanning of faces in autism. J. Autism Dev. Disord. 32(4), 249–261 (2002)

8. Falck-Ytter, T., von Hofsten, C.: How special is social looking in ASD: a review. Prog. Brain Res. **189**, 209–222 (2011)
9. Speer, L.L., Cook, A.E., McMahon, W.M., Clark, E.: Face processing in children with autism: effects of stimulus contents and type. Autism **11**(3), 265–277 (2007)
10. Hochreiter, S., Schmidhuber, J.: Long short-term memory. Neural comput. **9**(8), 1735–1780 (1997)

Automatic Detector of Abnormal EEG
for Preterm Infants

Nisrine Jrad[1]([✉]), Daniel Schang[2], Pierre Chauvet[1], Sylvie Nguyen The Tich[3], Bassam Daya[4], and Marc Gibaud[3]

[1] UCO-LARIS-UNAM, 3 place Andre-Leroy, BP 10808, 49008 Angers, France
nisrine.jrad@uco.fr
[2] ESEO Tech-UNAM, 10 Bld Jean Jeanneteau, 49009 Angers Cedex, France
[3] CHU-LARIS-UNAM, 4 rue Larrey, 49000 Angers, France
[4] Institute of Technology, Lebanese University, Saida, Lebanon

Abstract. Many of preterm babies suffer from neural disorders caused by birth complications. Hence, early prediction of neural disorders, in preterm infants, is extremely crucial for neuroprotective intervention. In this scope, the goal of this research was to propose an automatic way to study preterm babies Electroencephalograms (EEG). EEG were pre-processed and a time series of standard deviation was computed. These series were thresholded to detect Inter Burst Intervals (IBI). Features were extracted from bursts and IBI and were then classified as Abnormal or Normal using a Multiple Linear Regression. The method was successfully validated on a corpus of 100 infants with no early indication of brain injury. It was also implemented with a user-friendly interface using Java.

Keywords: Automatic EEG analysis · Inter Burst Interval Detection
Feature extraction · Multiple Linear Regression · Preterm infants

1 Introduction

Recent studies reported that 1 million preterm infants, among 15 millions born prematurely per year, were dead [1]. Unfortunately, many of the survived babies suffered from lifetime disabilities like visual and auditory problems, learning difficulties, etc. To avoid these disabilities, it is crucial to diagnose, prognose, and treat preterm born babies as quickly and as accurately as possible [2,3]. Usually, preterm babies receive a special attention provided by neonatal intensive care units. Intensive care units monitor babies brain activities through non-invasive Electroencephalogram (EEG) recordings. In preterm infants, EEG is physiologically constituted by an alternation of bursts of activity and periods of suppression called Inter Burst Interval (IBI) (Fig. 1). The proportion and duration of IBI vary according to the sleep stages (more prolonged in the calm sleep) and according to the term of birth (more prolonged in premature babies).

In everyday clinical practice, the EEG analysis is still done visually which leads to several difficulties. First, physicians accustomed to the analysis of EEG

© ICST Institute for Computer Sciences, Social Informatics and Telecommunications Engineering 2018
M. U. Ahmed et al. (Eds.): HealthyIoT 2017, LNICST 225, pp. 82–87, 2018.
https://doi.org/10.1007/978-3-319-76213-5_12

of very preterm infants are rare, causing delays in the interpretation of EEG tracings. Besides, visual analysis are subjective. Furthermore, in small hospitals, the expertise is often not available. Therefore, it is highly crucial to automate the physician's EEG analysis. Several researches tried to automatize bursts detection and the occurrence of seizures of full-term babies. For instance, authors of [4], proposed a method to discriminate between seizure and non-seizure EEG epochs of full-term babies. However, EEG characteristics vary a lot between preterm infants and full-term infants [5]. Few numbers of studies tackled the problem of identifying abnormal EEG of preterm infants. In the scope of automatic EEG analysis for prematurely newborns, we can quote the work presented in [3]. The authors proposed a method for automated burst detection based on *line length*, which is a running sum of the absolute differences between all consecutive samples within a predefined window [6].

Our motivation is to complete these studies by an automatic analysis of preterm EEG so as to detect abnormal brain activities, like an expert would have interpreted EEG. This allows to prioritize EEG that should be urgently analyzed by neurologist. To the best of our knowledge, there was no research addressing this task. Our method consisted on preprocessing data; EEG was filtered, using a band-stop IIR filter and smoothed using a moving average window. After, IBI were detected by thresholding standard deviation of preprocessed EEG. Relevant features were extracted from IBI and bursts and were then classified using a Multiple Linear Regression. Performance measures were evaluated using Areas Under the ROC Curves (AUC, [7,8]). The proposed method was validated on a cohort of 100 preterm babies, with no severe brain injuries.

The paper is outlined as follows: Sect. 2 describes the database that was collected. Section 3 accounts for the method. Section 4 shows results. Finally a conclusion is drawn.

2   Materials

EEG signals from 100 preterm babies were recorded in the neonatal intensive care unit of neuropediatric department of the University Hospital of Angers in France. This monitoring was part of the usual clinical follow up of premature babies. All babies legal representative gave informed consent for participation in research studies. EEG was recorded, with a sampling rate of 256 Hz, using the Alliance (Nicolet Biomedical) recording system with reduced neonatal montages of 8 to 11 adapted scalp electrodes according to the head size. Electrodes were placed according to the international 10–20 system. No hardware filter was used in the acquisition procedure, except the high-pass filter with 0.1 Hz as a cut-off frequency classically used to remove the offset of the baseline.

A total of 416 EEG recordings of 30 to 45 min durations were performed between January 1, 2003 and December 31 2004. All the 100 infants had less than 35 weeks of gestation. Each infant had between 1 to 7 EEG recordings resulting into the 416 EEG recordings. The 416 EEG were reviewed by a neuro-pediatrician and classified as normal, abnormal and doubtful. This classification

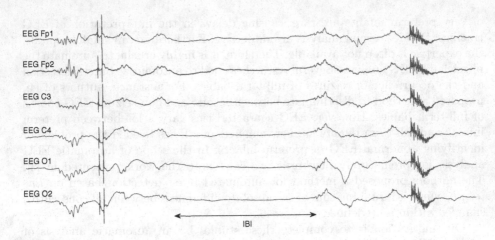

Fig. 1. An IBI example.

has been achieved through a careful visual analysis: EEG was considered as normal if the background activity (in relation to the gestation age) was normal and no abnormal features on the EEG were seen. The abnormal EEG were those who showed excessive discontinuity with maximal IBI duration above 50% of the maximal value (in relation to the gestation age), seizures, positive rolandic sharp waves of more than 2 per minute. 100 EEG recordings were considered as doubtful and were rejected. Finally, for the 316 kept EEG, the visual eye inspection gave 274 normal (88.77%, 31.04 ± 2.13 weeks of gestation) and 42 abnormal (11.23%, 30.01 ± 2.19 weeks of gestation) EEG. An example of abnormal EEG is illustrated in Fig. 1.

3   Methods

3.1   Problem Statement

Let $s(t)$ denote the EEG signal of N samples recorded in a given electrode. This signal essentially contains background activity where abnormal activities (IBI with discontinuity, seizures, rolandic sharp waves, etc.) may appear. The problem, addressed in this paper, consists of detecting the IBI and then classifying EEG into normal or abnormal. Automatic detection of abnormal EEG was done in four steps: preprocessing, IBI detection, feature extraction and EEG classification. In this section, each of these steps was detailed.

3.2   Preprocessing

For each electrode, raw EEG signal $s(t)$ was band-stop filtered at 50 Hz with a notch second order Butterworth IIR filter, so as to obtain a filtered signal

$s_{BP}(t)$ where the 50 Hz power supply frequency was removed. Then, $s_{BP}(t)$ was smoothed by computing the moving average over a window of width ω_1:

$$s_{MA}[n] = \frac{1}{\omega_1} \sum_{k=n-\omega_1/2}^{n+\omega_1/2} s_{BP}[k], n = 1, \ldots, N \tag{1}$$

3.3 IBI Detection

To detect IBI, standard deviation of signal $s_{MA}(t)$ was computed and thresholded like in [9]. Indeed, standard deviation was computed on sliding windows of size ω_2 with an overlap of ω_3 samples ($\omega_3 < \omega_2$) as following:

$$\nu^2[n] = \frac{1}{\omega_2 - 1} \sum_{k=n\omega_3}^{n\omega_3+\omega_2-1} s_{MA}^2[k] - \frac{1}{\omega_2(\omega_2-1)} \left(\sum_{k=n\omega_3}^{n\omega_3+\omega_2-1} s_{MA}[k] \right)^2, n = 1, \ldots, N \tag{2}$$

Successive standard deviation series with values below a threshold V_T (in μV) and longer than 1 s in duration were detected and delineated by an onset and an offset boundary limit markers. Consecutive detections less than 0.5 s apart were grouped together and considered as the same IBI. Finally, only IBI present across all EEG electrodes and longer than 1 s were kept.

3.4 Feature Extraction

For each EEG electrode, a vector of 13 features was extracted as following:

1. Number of IBI: nb_IBI,
2. Total duration of IBI, defined as the sum of all IBI durations: tot_IBI (seconds),
3. Percentage of IBI in the EEG: $P\_IBI(\%) = \frac{tot\_IBI}{EEG\_duration}$,
4. Duration of the longest IBI: Max_IBI (seconds),
5. The maximum of IBI percentage in the EEG, $P\_Max\_IBI(\%) = \frac{Max\_IBI}{EEG\_duration}$,
6. The mean duration of IBI, defined as the sum of the IBI durations divided by the number of IBI: $Mean\_IBI$ (seconds),
7. Number of bursts: nb_B,
8. Total duration of the bursts calculated as the sum of all bursts durations, tot_B (seconds),
9. Percentage of bursts in the EEG, $P\_B(\%) = \frac{tot\_B}{EEG\_duration}$,
10. The duration of the longest burst: Max_B (seconds),
11. The maximum of bursts percentage in the EEG: $P\_Max\_B(\%) = \frac{Max\_B}{EEGduration}$,
12. The mean duration of the bursts calculated as the sum of the bursts durations divided by the number of bursts, $Mean\_B$ (seconds),
13. The gestational age of the newborn at the time of the EEG examination: Age_EEG in weeks.

3.5 Multiple Linear Regression

Extracted features formed a set of vectors $x_m \in \mathbb{R}^d, m = 1, \ldots, M$ with M the total number of EEG electrodes and $d = 13$ the number of extracted features. The entire data set was written as $\{(x_1, y_1), \ldots, (x_m, y_m), \ldots, (x_M, y_M)\}$ with class labels $y_m \in \{+1, -1\}$ for Abnormal and Normal EEG respectively. Learning a Multiple Regression classifier consisted on finding a function f:

$$f : \mathbb{R}^d \longrightarrow \mathbb{R}$$

$$x \longmapsto f(x) = \sum_{i=1}^{d} w_i x_i + b \tag{3}$$

with $w \in \mathbb{R}^d$ is the slope and $b \in \mathbb{R}$ is the intercept of the function f. The predicted class is then given by the sign of f. Hence, we have to compute $\alpha = \begin{bmatrix} w \\ b \end{bmatrix} \in \mathbb{R}^{d+1}$ minimizing the quadratic error:

$$\min_{\alpha \in \mathbb{R}^{d+1}} \|\epsilon\|^2 = \min_{\alpha \in \mathbb{R}^{d+1}} \|y - \mathbf{X}\alpha\|^2 \tag{4}$$

with $y = \begin{bmatrix} y_1 \\ \vdots \\ y_m \\ \vdots \\ y_M \end{bmatrix}$ and $\mathbf{X} = \begin{bmatrix} x_{1,1} & x_{1,2} & \ldots x_{1,d} & 1 \\ \vdots & \vdots & \vdots & \vdots \\ x_{m,1} & x_{m,2} & \ldots x_{m,d} & 1 \\ \vdots & \vdots & \vdots & \vdots \\ x_{M,1} & x_{M,2} & \ldots x_{M,d} & 1 \end{bmatrix}$. The solution was given by $\hat{\alpha} = (\mathbf{X}^T \mathbf{X})^{-1} \mathbf{X}^T y$.

4 Results and Discussion

Experiments on EEG data set, described in Sect. 2, were conducted to evaluate performance of the proposed method. Performance were quantitatively analyzed using the Receiver Operating Characteristic (ROC) curves [7]. The ROC curve is a parametric plot representing sensitivity as a function of specificity for different thresholds. Area Under the ROC curve, AUC, was computed for a handy representation of results [7]. The whole data set was resampled, using a 5-cross validation, into training and testing sets on a per class basis.

Mean comparison statistical tests of Abnormal versus Normal features revealed that these distributions have different means with p-values under 0.01. Experimental results showed that Multiple Linear Regression estimated on temporal features can detect accurately abnormal EEG. The optimal threshold V_T was of $23\,\mu\text{V}$. Detection of an abnormal preterm infant EEG reached a sensitivity of $85.83\% \pm 15.97$ and a specificity of $74.14\% \pm 15.97$ with an AUC of $80.00\% \pm 0.08$. Thus, if the automatic detection considered that an EEG is abnormal, it must be interpreted primarily by the doctor to undergo more medical examinations such as an MRI (Magnetic Resonance Imaging) scanner, an expensive test that can not be done routinely. Moreover, due to the high sensitivity, an EEG classified as normal does not need to be interpreted urgently by the neurologist.

It is worthy to note that performance were achieved on a set of 416 EEG after rejecting 100 doubtful EEG. It will be interesting to learn a classifier that automatically labels these suspicious as doubtful. The correlation of our results with the outcome at 2 years was not done because infants who were clinically diagnosed as pathological and treated had a chance of recovering. Finally, the proposed method was implemented, using java, in a user-friendly interface designed to inspect detection results and test different parameters, if needed.

5 Conclusion

This study presented a software for automatic detection of abnormal Electroencephalograms (EEG) of preterm infants. The method consisted on detecting Inter Burst Intervals, extracting features from EEG and classifying them into normal or abnormal EEG. Experimental results illustrated the efficiency of the proposed method in terms of sensitivity and specificity. These findings are very promising and encourage further researches that may enhance detection of abnormal EEG.

References

1. Howson, C., Kinney, M., McDougall, J.L.L.: Born too soon: preterm birth matters. Reprod. Health **10**(1). https://doi.org/10.1186/1742-4755-10-S1-S1
2. Deburchgraeve, W., Cherian, P., Vos, M.D., Swarte, R., Blok, J., Visser, G., Govaert, P., Huffel, S.V.: Automated neonatal seizure detection mimicking a human observer reading EEG. Clin. Neurophysiol. **119**(11), 2447–2454 (2008)
3. Koolen, N., Jansen, K., Vervisch, J., Matic, V., Vos, M.D., Naulaers, G., Huffel, S.V.: Line length as a robust method to detect high-activity envents: automated burst detection in premature EEG recordings. Clin. Neurophysiol. **125**(10), 1985–1994 (2014)
4. Temko, A., Thomas, E., Marnane, W., Lightbody, G., Boylan, G.: EEG-based neonatal seizure detection with support vector machines. Clin. Neurophysiol. **122**(3), 464–473 (2010)
5. Joseph, J., Lesevre, N., Dreyfus-Brisac, C.: Spatio-temporal organization of EEG in premature infants and full-term new-borns. Electroencephalogr. Clin. Neurophysiol. **40**(2), 153–168 (1976)
6. Esteller, R., Echauz, J., Tcheng, T., Litt, B., Pless, B.: Line length: an efficient feature for seizure onset detection. In: Proceedings of the 23rd IEEE EMBS International Conference (2001)
7. Hanley, J., McNeil, B.: The meaning and use of the area under a receiver operating characteristic (ROC) curve. Radiology **143**, 29–36 (1982)
8. Fawcett, T.: An introduction to ROC analysis. Pattern Recogn. Lett. Spec. Issue ROC Anal. **27**, 861–874 (2006)
9. Chauvet, P., Tich, S.N.T., Schang, D., Clement, A.: Evaluation of automatic feature detection algorithms in EEG: application to interburst intervals. Comput. Biol. Med. **54**, 61–71 (2014)

Check for
updates

Non-invasive Analytics Based Smart System
for Diabetes Monitoring

M. Saravanan[1(✉)] and R. Shubha[2]

[1] Ericsson Research, Ericsson India Global Services Pvt. Ltd., Chennai, India
m.saravanan@ericsson.com
[2] School of Electronics Engineering, VIT University, Chennai, India
shubharavi20@gmail.com

Abstract. Wearable devices have made it possible for health providers to monitor a patient's health remotely using actuators, sensors and other mobile communication devices. Internet of Things for Medical Devices is poised to revolutionize the functioning of the healthcare industry by providing an environment where the patient data is transmitted via a gateway onto a secure cloud based platforms for storage, aggregation and analytics. This paper proposes new set of wearable devices - a smart neck band, smart wrist band and a pair of smart socks - to continuously monitor the condition of diabetic patients. These devices consist of different sensors working in tandem form a network that reports food intake, heart rate, skin moisture, ambient temperature, walking patterns and weight gain/loss. The devices with the aid of controllers send all the sensor values as a packet via Bluetooth to the Mobile App. With the help of Machine Learning algorithm, we have predicted the change in patient status and alert them.

Keywords: Diabetes monitoring · Non-invasive method · Sensors and devices
PSO algorithm · Mobile app

1 Introduction

Diabetes Mellitus kills and disables, impoverishes families, imposes a huge economic burden on governments and business and overwhelms health systems [1]. The healthcare industry is interested in meeting two important goals in a cost-effective way by improving clinical outcomes and enhancing patient care. In order to improve clinical outcomes, real-time measurement and management of illnesses are considered as important features. Providing a better quality of life and user experience to patients is critical to enhancing patient care. IOT in Medical Devices, also known as IOT-MD, promises a cost-effective way to achieve these two goals of the healthcare industry. Connected healthcare programs utilize scarce resources to provide an improved quality of care which leads to better clinical outcomes. Measurable benefits of connected medical devices include reduction in mortality rates, fewer clinic visits, reduced emergency and hospital admissions, including reduction in bed days of care and length of stay in hospitals. Remote monitoring of patients leads to more effective and timely treatment and also it leads to a better management of healthcare [2]. In addition,

© ICST Institute for Computer Sciences, Social Informatics and Telecommunications Engineering 2018
M. U. Ahmed et al. (Eds.): HealthyIoT 2017, LNICST 225, pp. 88–98, 2018.
https://doi.org/10.1007/978-3-319-76213-5_13

patients (and their relatives) are empowered by getting greater visibility into their actual health conditions, enabling them to play an active role in controlling and influencing their treatment.

Wearable technology, unlike the traditional invasive mechanisms provides continuous monitoring of diabetic people. Basically, there are two ways to provide solutions for the diabetic patients i.e., traditional methods which are invasive in nature and the other one is the more commonly used non-invasive method. Recently, Nanotechnology has come to the fore and contributed in introducing new medical devices in both invasive and non-invasive methods which provide solutions to those suffering from diabetes mellitus. It has paved a way for the invention of Nano Tattoos as well as Nano-based glucose sensors which are used to monitor the glucose level without the need of taking blood samples often [3, 4]. The application of IoT to such Nano-based devices which includes Nanocapsules [5] made the diabetes monitoring even easier. These IoT devices gather patient information from time to time and perform the required processing to provide the information to the patient as well as the doctor/care takers. When addressing such global health issues, one has to provide an end-to-end solution which is cost effective and lasts over a period of time. Bearing all the required features in mind a new non-invasive solution is proposed to monitor diabetic people in real-time.

In the proposed work, a solution is based on three wearable devices, a Smart watch, Smart socks and a Smart neck band which monitors symptoms like frequency of food and water intake, heart rate, skin moisture, ambient temperature, walking patterns and weight. These symptoms are crucial for any diabetic patient and thus, with the data gathered, a stochastic optimization technique is applied on all three devices readings to predict the sudden increase/decrease in glucose level of the patient and thus notify them ahead of time to prevent complication due to diabetes and prevent any fatal effect. Particle swarm Optimization (PSO) [6], a computational method is used here to improve the quality of the solution for real-time prediction. Our system can able to store data for millions of patients to perform analysis in real time, ultimately promoting an evidence-based medicine system.

2   Related Works

In today's world, many devices are available which work with specific methods to monitor diabetic patients. All methods are efficient enough to detect the glucose level but they do lack in certain criteria like performing prediction on real-time streaming data obtained from the sensors attached with the patient's body and provide them with alerts. There are two methods used for diabetes monitoring i.e. invasive and non-invasive. Invasive method uses pricking mechanism that uses blood samples for the detection of glucose level. The existing invasive mechanism for glucose monitoring are Glucose-meter [7] and Gmate Smart [8] which are medical devices that are used for determining the approximate concentration of glucose in the blood. It uses either sensor strips or devices that require blood from pricking in order to determine the glucose level. The detected level is notified to the patient with the help of an app specific to that device. The app based existing monitoring system includes ShugaTrak [9] and Glucose Buddy [9]. Using the app, people with diabetes can easily communicate their blood glucose levels to their loved ones. The apps also incorporate diary for diet, medication, and exercise habit logging. They aim to close the gap between patients and healthcare providers by including the option to have glucose readings sent via e-mail to the patient's medical team. The existing Nano-based non-invasive mechanisms include Nanosensors [4] and Nano-ink Tattoos [4]. The Nano-ink Tattoos are injected into the skin, much like tattoo dye to monitor an individual's blood-sugar level. As the glucose level increases, the "tattoo" fluoresces under an infrared light, telling a diabetic patient whether or not they need an insulin shot following a meal. Smart Sox [10] are designed to identify locations in the foot as well as ranges of motion that could lead to problems. The socks use fiber optics and sensors to monitor changing pressures in the patient's feet. Artificial or Bionic Pancreas [11] is another device in which a signal is transmitted wirelessly every 5 min from a glucose monitor under the patient's skin to a smartphone app. The app will then calculate the amount of insulin or glucagon needed to balance blood glucose, automatically sending a signal to the pumps carried by the user in order to administer the required dose via a tube. CGM [12] is connected to a transmitter that sends the information via wireless radio frequency to a monitoring and display device. The device can detect and notify you if your glucose is reaching a high or low limit. Smart Watches are the wearables that record parameters like heart rate, step count, sleep quality and many such parameters are needed for the monitoring and have to be recorded for a diabetic person [13].

All these existing systems have their own advantages but they do not provide a solution in terms of real-time prediction and early symptom identification [14]. This paper therefore aims at overcoming this limitation to provide end-to-end system which measures all diabetic required features. Moreover, by running the prediction algorithm on the real-time data, the patient can be notified before their condition worsens, thereby decreasing the mortality rate of the human beings. This non-invasive solution when coupled with the real-time information assist in prediction using Particle Swarm Organization (PSO) and help to suggest suitable remedies to diabetic patients is considered as a good model for continuous monitoring and prevention of complications to diabetic patient. In the proposed system, PSO act as a data optimization model in predicting the present status and any serious implications of the diabetes patient from the data collected on three different wearable devices.

3 Proposed Solution

In the proposed solution, we have designed three wearables which include a smart neck band, smart wrist band and smart footwear (or socks) for monitoring the patients and to understand their present condition. The smart neck band comprises of vibration sensors and an array of strain gauges to measure the frequency of food and water intake. Smart wrist band comprises of moisture sensor, temperature sensor and heart rate sensor that provides data about the sweat rate, ambient temperature and the heart rate of the patient. The smart footwear includes pressure sensors and weight sensor which is helpful in determining fatigue and weight. Foot analysis is performed to determine the walking pattern of the patients that gives details regarding the unhealed wounds and other foot complications with few exceptions. All the three modules communicate with a wireless Bluetooth module which transmits the data to the patient's Mobile Phone (or other personal assistants) which acts as a gateway to upload the data to the Health Cloud. By applying relevant Machine Learning and Statistical techniques, the stored data will be analyzed and suitable steps be suggested based on the prediction so as to minimize the effect of complication. Communication layer (Information Processing) present in proposed architecture will be capable enough to send suitable notifications regarding the patient's situation to the concerned doctor at an early stage to avoid the complications in patient's health. We will first explain the details of devices as provided in Fig. 1 and the execution of devices will be explained through a flow chart.

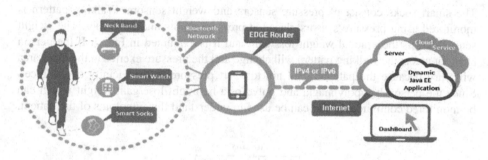

Fig. 1. Overview of the proposed system

3.1 Smart Neck Band

The device consists of a smart neck band which basically monitors two important parameters which are the frequency of food and water intake (polyphagia and polydipsia). The data from the sensor is obtained then passed to the mobile application using a Bluetooth connection then later forwarded to cloud for the purpose of analysis.

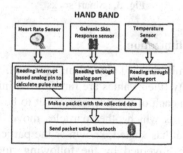

Fig. 2. Smart wrist band

3.2   Smart Wrist Band

It comprises of a smart watch that monitors the heart rate, skin moisture and ambient temperature. Temperature sensor, optical heart rate sensor and galvanic skin response sensor are used to monitor the above mentioned parameters. Temperature is monitored to know the altitude, as the altitude plays an important role in the blood glucose level, when there is an increase in blood sugar level the heart rate keeps fluctuating. Similarly, the skin moisture also varies for diabetic people and data collected from all the connected sensors will be sent it to the mobile application via a Bluetooth so that the data is forwarded to the cloud for storage and prediction. The details are illustrated in Fig. 2.

3.3   Smart Socks

The smart socks consist of pressure sensors and weight sensors. Walking pattern is monitored using pressure sensors placed at pressure points under the foot. The weight sensor detects the gradual weight loss/gain and it is explained in Fig. 3. If the person has foot ulcers the walking pattern will change and the pressure exerted at the ulcer area will vary because the patients tend not to exert pressure in the vicinity of the ulcer. Since the person has polyphagia and polydipsia he might lose/gain weight which can be monitored continuously and can be used to understand the symptoms of the patient.

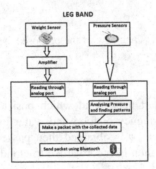

Fig. 3. Smart socks

3.4   Particle Swarm Optimization

In the Particle swarm optimization [6] algorithm, each particle belonging to a swarm, has a position and a velocity (their values are randomized initially). The position with the highest fitness score, in each of the iteration, is set to be the entire swarm's global best (gbest) position, towards which other particles move. In addition, each particle keeps its best position that it has visited, known as the particle's personal best (pbest). The particle dynamics are governed by the following rules which update particle positions and velocities:

$$v_i = wv_i + c1r1(\, pbest,\, i - x_i) + c2r2(gbest - x_i) \tag{1}$$

$$x_i = x_i + v_i \tag{2}$$

where x_i is the current position of particle i, pbest is the best position attained by particle i, gbest is the swarm's global best position, v_i is the velocity of particle i, w is a random inertia weight, c1 and c2 are spring constants and r1 and r2 are random numbers between 0 and 1. In this paper, the implementation of PSO is slightly modified and applied to the list of features extracted from three wearables and different embedded sensors to understand the present status of the diabetes patient.

The proposed system is developed with very minimal cost and provides accurate readings with sensors to solve the global health issue of diabetes. This solution can help reduce the world's health expenditure and can help improve the economy i.e. the solution is cost effective and thereby all classes of people can afford such a solution. The main complication of the disease is laid on monitoring, which is overcome by using wearable technologies made with different sensors. When a person with diabetes is continuously monitored, their condition will be under constant surveillance so that any adverse consequence can be prevented in advance. It also predicts the glucose level based on the symptoms exhibited from day-to-day. The data obtained from wearables will be stored on the cloud for future analysis of the patient's condition. The data can thus be accessed by both the doctor as well as the patient.

After processing the data obtained from the three wearables, the coefficient for all three modules is calculated and that is given as the input to Particle swarm optimization (PSO) algorithm. PSO is then applied to predict the present status of diabetes for a specific person. The application of PSO to the list of extracted features of three devices is as follows.

At each time step, the pieces of variable information a given particle (wearable) knows and it can transmit are:

- The current value x_i and the corresponding function value.
- Best position found so far, *pbest* and the corresponding function value.
- Previous position (to estimate its improvement).

Each wearable is assigned a weight along three different axes representing its coefficient. The axes mentioned here are related to the inputs from three wearables and its embedded sensors. Each and every wearable is assigned a position on each axis based on their values in any of the methods. The sum of weights on all the three axes gives the current value of the wearable. Features such as food intake, heart rate, skin moisture, ambient temperature, walking patterns and weight gain/loss are also used to calculate the position of the wearable presence in the model. The wearable's rank is then updated using Eq. (2) which is based on their value. The particles (wearables) are then ranked based on their closeness to the gbest of the swarm. That is clearly explained in the pseudocode given here

Pseudo Code:

```
For each particle {
   Initialize particle
}
Do until maximum iterations or minimum error criteria {
   For each particle
   {
       Calculate Data fitness value
       If the fitness value is better than pBest
       {
           Set pBest = current fitness value
       }
       If pBest is better than gBest
       {
          Set gBest = pBest
       }
   }
   For each particle
   {
       Calculate particle Velocity
       Use gBest and Velocity to update particle Data
   }
}
```

Equation (2) has been used to rank the wearables contribution using the redefined features. Here x_i is the wearable value in the list, v_i is the wearable weight factor which measures of the closeness of the wearable involved to measure the seriousness of diabetes. Pbest, is the wearable best position, gbest, is the best position obtained for the swarm, w is a random inertia weight with value 0.1, c1 and c2 are spring constants with values 1 and r1 and r2 are random numbers with values vary from 0 to 1. The final contribution of wearables is displayed in a ranked manner. Based on the contribution, a prediction is made related to the condition of diabetes of a patient which will be informed to them through Mobile app.

The flowchart shown in Fig. 4 describes the working model of the entire system in which the data is being read from Smart neck band, threshold is set for the module and relevant coefficient value of the module is calculated. Similarly, the embedded sensor values from the other two wearables – the wrist band and socks are read, the threshold for the modules is set and their respective coefficients are recorded. The coefficients relevant to various features will be obtained and these values are inputted to the PSO algorithm to predict consequence of the changes in glucose levels. Here all three device feature inputs will be attracted to the central node which predicts the real consequences. If the respective module's value exceeds the set threshold, individual sensor values are checked to see if their threshold exceeded and thereby the glucose level has increased

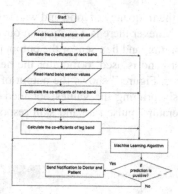

Fig. 4. Flow chart of the system

over a period of time. When the algorithm provides a positive prediction then alert notification will be sent to the patient's mobile.

4 Results and Discussion

The System mainly focuses on supervising the symptoms that a diabetic person exhibits using various sensors embedded in the neck band, wrist band and socks. From the output of neck band, we get to know the food intake quantity so that one can control their blood sugar by managing their diet. Smart socks will specify the possible area where foot ulcer can occur and hence the user can start medication for that area. With the data obtained we can know the current level as well as expected future levels based on the current levels. These results are shown via the mobile app so that the patient can ascertain an increase or decrease in their glucose levels. We have conducted few clinical trials and the results of three different devices sample values are provided here as a result for our experiments.

Smart socks contain pressure sensor to detect the walking pattern depending on the pressure exerted on pressure points. Figure 5 shows the output of pressure sensors. The pressure sensors are placed at the four pressure points of the leg, the spikes in the image describe that even pressure is applied on the pressure points.

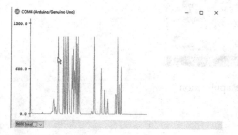

Fig. 5. Output of smart socks device

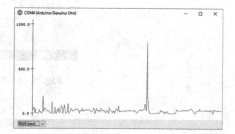

Fig. 6. Output of vibration and flex

Smart neck band detects the frequency of food and water intake. Figure 6 shows the output of neck module i.e. whenever there is a motion on our jaw as well as movement on our throat detected by vibration and flex sensor the output produced would be a high amplitude spike. Smart wrist band is used to monitor the heart rate, moisture content and temperature using sensors. Figure 7 shows the output of smart hand module. The serial monitor is continuously printing the values obtained from the sensor of wrist band such as ambient temperature, pulse rate and skin response.

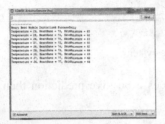

Fig. 7. Output of smart wrist band device

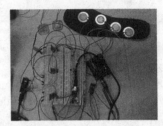

Fig. 8. Interfacing three modules together

The combined circuitry and placement of sensors of all the three modules are made. Figure 8 shows the interfacing of all three wearable modules with the controller and a Bluetooth module to provide the required data. In order to make the mobile function as a gateway, a user friendly mobile app is designed. Figure 9 shows the android app that is developed for the application which has the slot for all three wearables. It will help the patient view his vital parameters at any point in time. The App not only display the vitals but will also have the meal count of the patient and will identify the ulcer location on his foot via the App.

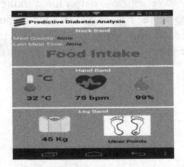

Fig. 9. Mobile application

Diabetes is a major burden to the economy of the world. Globally, 12% of the health expenditure and USD 1330 (ID 1478) per person is anticipated to be spent on monitoring diabetes. Therefore, entire world requires a solution which is feasible, effective and affordable by the common public. From the results obtained for the solution, it's evident that the proposed technology satisfies all the criteria required. The sensors used are accurate and are of low cost. The sensor devices will last over a long period, unlike the disposable strips used in many techniques. The overall manufacturing cost is less and hence even the common public can afford it. As a result, the global expenditure spent per person will be minimized. A system which satisfies all the above constraints is designed and its effectiveness is been proved. Many of the existing systems fail to satisfy the above criteria, all of which are equally important for a healthcare solution. The solution mainly concentrates on providing an end-to-end non-invasive solution for diabetic people using the implementation of IoT-MD and wearable technology while being cost effective. The data from three wearbles is obtained and processing is done to provide the effective output. After the sufficient clinical trials, we found that our solution gives promising outcomes and strongly acknowledge the usefulness of new technology. We also found that the total cost of the entire prototype will be approximately around USD 150 per person.

5 Conclusion

The sudden rise in the number of diabetic patients all over the world and the high cost of monitoring systems calls for innovation in the field of IoT-MD. The application of IOT sensors in diabetics monitoring helped in figuring out the solution for designing wearables using compact sensor devices for the Smart neck band which makes the device weigh less and thereby not be of any hindrance to the patient who uses it. The above proposed system monitors diabetes from the point of view of symptoms a diabetic patient exhibits, that continuously monitor glucose levels using wearable technology. It also emphasizes the advantage of using wearable technology so that a person can know his/her condition at any moment and will get notified about their present status via the mobile app to take precautionary measures to prevent any adverse effects. With further developments, the solution can even act as a patient's care taker as well as a doctor's assisting device.

References

1. https://www.idf.org/sites/default/files/Policy_Briefing_GlobalHealth.pdf
2. Jara, A.J., Zamora, M.A., Skarmeta, A.F.G.: An Internet of Things–Based Personal Device for Diabetes Therapy Management in Ambient Assisted Living (AAL). Springer, London (2011)
3. DiSanto, R.M., Subramanian, V., Gu, Z.: Recent advances in nanotechnology for diabetes treatment. Wiley Interdiscip. Rev. Nanomed. Nanobiotechnol. **7**(4), 548–564 (2015)
4. Cash, K.J., Clark, H.A.: Nanosensors and nanomaterials for monitoring glucose in diabetes. Trends Mol. Med. **16**(12), 584–593 (2010)

5. Mooranian, A., Negrulj, R., Takechi, R., Jamieson, E., Morahan, G., Al-Salami, H.: New biotechnological microencapsulating methodology utilizing individualized gradient-screened jet laminar flow techniques for pancreatic β-cell delivery: bile acids support cell energy-generating mechanisms. Mol. Pharm. **14**(8), 2711–2718 (2017)
6. Kirchsteiger, H., Jørgensen, J.B., Renard, E., del Re, L. (eds.): Prediction Methods for Blood Glucose Concentration. Springer, Cham (2016). https://doi.org/10.1007/978-3-319-25913-0
7. Gabbay, R.A.: Diabetes management key to health care solutions. Am. J. Manag. Care **20**, e72–e81 (2014)
8. http://www.mayoclinic.org/diseases-conditions/diabetes/expert-blog/blood-glucose-monitoring/bgp-20056564
9. https://www.diabetes.ie/smart-diabetes-technology-on-the-horizon/
10. Perrier, A., vuillerme, N., Luboz, V., Payan, Y.: Smart diabetic socks: embedded device for diabetic foot prevention. IRBM **35**(2) (2014)
11. Russell, S.J., El-Khatib, F.H., Sinha, M., Magyar, K.L., Katherine, N.P., McKeon, M., Goergen, L.G., Balliro, C., Hillard, M.A., Nathan, D.M., Damiano, E.R.: Outpatient glycemic control with a bionic pancreas in Type 1 diabetes. New Engl. J. Med. **371**, 313–325 (2014)
12. Tamborlane, W.V., Beck, R.W.: Continuos glucose monitoring and intensive treatment of Type 1 diabetes. The juvenile diabetes research foundation continuous glucose monitoring study group (2008)
13. Marling, C., Wiley, M., Bunescu, R., Shubrook, J., Schwartz, F.: Emerging applications for intelligent diabetes management. Assoc. Adv. Artif. Intell. **33**(2) (2017)
14. Tafa, Z., Pervetica, N., Karahoda, B.: An intelligent system for diabetes prediction. In: 4th Mediterranean Conference on Embedded Computing (MECO), 14–18 June 2015

Posters Track

Cloud-Based Data Analytics on Human Factor Measurement to Improve Safer Transport

Mobyen Uddin Ahmed[1(✉)], Shahina Begum[1],
Carlos Alberto Catalina[2], Lior Limonad[3], Bertil Hök[4],
and Gianluca Di Flumeri[5]

[1] School of Innovation, Design and Engineering,
Mälardalen University, 72123 Västerås, Sweden
{mobyen.ahmed, shahina.begum}@mdh.se
[2] ITCL, Polígono Industrial Villalonquéjar c/López Bravo,
70, 09001 Burgos, Spain
carlos.catalina@itcl.es
[3] Smart Wearable and IoT Solutions, IBM Research, Haifa, Israel
LIORLI@il.ibm.com
[4] Hök Instrument AB, Flottiljgatan 49, 72131 Västerås, Sweden
bertil.hok@hokinstrument.com
[5] Cognitive States in Operative Environment, BrainSigns,
Via Sesto Celere, 7/C, Rome, Italy
gianluca.diflumeri@brainsigns.com

Abstract. Improving safer transport includes individual and collective behavioural aspects and their interaction. A system that can monitor and evaluate the human cognitive and physical capacities based on human factor measurement is often beneficial to improve safety in driving condition. However, analysis and evaluation of human factor measurement i.e. demographics, behaviour and physiology in real-time is challenging. This paper presents a methodology for cloud-based data analysis, categorization and metrics correlation in real-time through a H2020 project called SimuSafe. Initial implementation of this methodology shows a step-by-step approach which can handle huge amount of data with variation and verity in the cloud.

Keywords: SimuSafe · Safer transport · Data-analysis · Big data
Human factor

1 Introduction

As it can be found in [1, 2], there are around 90% of road-traffic crashes caused by driver error (i.e. as inattention, loss of vigilance, mental under/overload) and unsafe behavior (i.e. inadequate training or lack of experience). Improving road safety includes understanding the individual, collective and interaction behaviour of drivers and pedestrians. A system that can monitor and evaluate the human cognitive and physical capacities based on human factor measurements is often beneficial to improve safety in driving condition and, more in general, in the whole transportation domain [14]. Due to increased data volume, real time data acquisition and heterogeneous

© ICST Institute for Computer Sciences, Social Informatics and Telecommunications Engineering 2018
M. U. Ahmed et al. (Eds.): HealthyIoT 2017, LNICST 225, pp. 101–106, 2018.
https://doi.org/10.1007/978-3-319-76213-5_14

sources data analytics i.e., data processing, analyzing and visualizing is becoming a challenging task. Several authors have focused on data analytics platform based on ongoing challenges [3, 4]. Most of these challenges are about real-time processing, handling of massive data, storage capacity, processing speed and so on. Companies like Google and Amazon have been trying to overcome these challenges using Hadoop or similar exiting data systems [5, 6].

This paper presents a methodology for cloud-based data analysis, categorization and metrics correlation in real-time through a H2020 project called SimuSafe[1]. The goal of SimuSafe is to identify behavioural models of drivers and pedestrians in a real traffic environment, implemented within traffic simulators with controllable settings, by applying artificial intelligence, virtual reality and data science methodologies. The proposed approach presented here shows the possibility to handle, process and analyze large amount of demographics, behavioural and physiological data with various variations coming both in offline and in real-time. Here, the proposed approach is implemented in IBM Bluemix cloud platform where the data analysis will be conducted in three Phases: (1) Information fusion and data abstraction, (2) Data mining and knowledge discovery and (3) Learning, reasoning and model creation.

2 System Overview

The data analytics will comprise with a data storage infrastructure to gather all relevant data (actor model states, user, cognitive and behavioural assessment data and annotations). This infrastructure will be integrated in IBM Bluemix cloud platform, further processing will be performed in the Data Analysis Server as presented in Fig. 1.

IBM Streaming and Predictive Analytics[2] from the platform will be employed to pre-filtering raw data sent to the Data Analysis server, for the real-time identification of events of interest and characteristic data patterns to be translated into components of the Actor Model. At the end of the analysis cycle, the correlation of relevant descriptors, patterns and states from the Actor model will be determined quantitatively, so responsible factors can be translated to high/low risk metric indices and used for calculation. Additionally, this data analysis will determine the cross-correlation and interdependency of data descriptor within the actor model. Tracing the effects and relations between the actor model components is essential since not all sensors are presented in Naturalistic Driving conditions (i.e. biometric data such as EEG, BVP, etc.). This approach will allow the computation of the actor model and risk metrics with a sensor subset, effectively removing the need of tests with a high degree of sensorization in later stages.

---

[1] www.simusafe.eu

[2] https://console.bluemix.net/catalog/?category=data

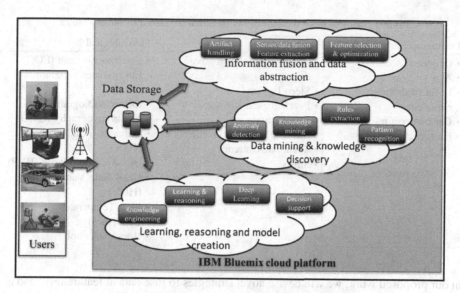

Fig. 1. Cloud-based data analytics approach

3 Materials and Method

The project is going to use three research cycles that will allow to reproduce and refine the model and metric in each cycle based on the measurements collected both considering Naturalistic Driving (ND), Controlled Environment (CE) and Simulation Driving Tests (SD). There will be two test groups preforming the test, constituted by pedestrian and both two-wheels and car drivers, with young adults (18–24 years) and elderlies (50–70 years). Total test subjects are about 458, in 1st cycle 90, 2nd cycle 42 and 3rd cycle 326 across the Europe (i.e. Spain, Sweden, France, Italy, UK, Poland). The sensor measurements will be collected derived from the Human, Vehicle and Environment components, however, in this paper we only consider Human factors. Human factor measurement will be collected from the subjects and is organized in three classes: Demographics, Behavioural and Physiological data, as summarized in Table 1.

The proposed cloud-based data analysis on human factor measurement to obtain required performance works in three Phase: **Phase 1:** Information fusion and data abstraction, **Phase 2:** Data mining and knowledge discovery and **Phase 3:** Learning, reasoning and model creation.

In *Phase 1*, the data pre-processing will be performed based on a combination of statistical, machine leaning and signal processing methods and techniques. Here, a robust and scalable data cleaning strategy will be established based on domain-specific knowledge, which will include sub-processes like cleaning, filtering, sampling or/and normalization. Our previous work on data pre-processing [9] using both structured and unstructured data will serve as a basis for online automated data cleaning. Traditional feature extraction methods [7] will be adapted to handle scalability issues in the domain.

Table 1. Summary of measurements parameters related to human factor.

Demographics	Behavioural	Physiological
• Gender • Age • Level of driving experience • Car ownership • Frequency of driving	• Propensity for aggressive driving • Sleep Hygiene • Psychological stressors • Driving Style • Incident/Violation Occurrence • Situation Awareness • Stress	• Electrooculogram (EOG) • Electroencephalogram (EEG) • Electrocardiogram (ECG) • Electromyography (EMG) • Galvanic Skin Response (GSR) • Blood Volume Pulse (BVP) • Heart Rate Variability (HRV) • Skin Temperature • Eye Tracking • Breath Alcohol

In our proposed work, we will devise novel strategies to fuse data at feature level and as well as at data level considering a defined fusion mechanism [8].

In *Phase 2*, a combination of potential sequences in the learning and search procedure will be investigated. The similarity assessment in the time series will be done by measuring the distance between probability distributions in the time series data mining [10]. A combination of statistical model and fuzzy modeling algorithm will be applied to automatic addition/deletion of rules, as well as adjustment of the membership functions. A continuous learning procedure will be developed so as to keep the model constantly updated [12]. In addition, new mining methods to support the discovery of knowledge [12] will be developed (Fig. 2).

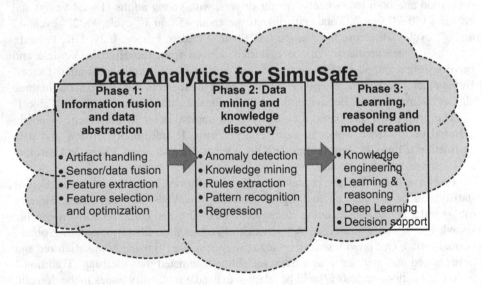

Fig. 2. Phases of the proposed data analytics approach in SimuSafe

In *Phase 3*, adaptation of dynamic knowledge representation approaches will be achieved by combining different artificial intelligence [12, 13] methods. This has a connection with Phase 2 as the data driven knowledge, rules and patterns will be considered as input. To provide decision support a hybrid approach will be applied utilizing different traditional machine learning algorithms, such as case-based reasoning, and clustering [11].

4 Summary

This paper proposed an approach for cloud-based data analysis, categorization and metrics correlation in real-time through a H2020 project called SimuSafe. The goal of the proposed approach shows the possibility to handle, process and analyze the Demographics, Behavioural and Physiological data in Big data contest. IBM Bluemix cloud platform is used with three parallel nodes where analytics phases are implemented. The phases are: (1) Information fusion and data abstraction, (2) Data mining and knowledge discovery and (3) Learning, reasoning and model creation. SimuSafe project is in its initial phase started in June 2017, several challenging works is ongoing.

Acknowledgments. The authors would like to acknowledge the project SimuSafe, the project has received funding from the European Union's Horizon 2020 research and innovation programme under grant agreement No 723386.

References

1. Elander, J., West, R., French, D.: Behavioural correlates of individual differences in road-traffic crash risk: an examination of methods and findings. Psychol. Bull. **113**(2), 279 (1993)
2. Feyer, A.M., Williamson, A., Friswell, R.: Balancing work and rest to combat driver fatigue: an investigation of two-up driving in Australia. Accid. Anal. Prevention **29**, 541–553 (1997)
3. Katal, A., Wazid, M., Goudar, R.H.: Big data: issues, challenges, tools and good practices. In: Contemporary Computing (IC3), pp. 404–409 (2013)
4. Zhang, D.: Inconsistencies in big data. In: 2013 12th IEEE International Conference on Cognitive Informatics & Cognitive Computing (ICCI*CC), pp. 61–67 (2013)
5. Rathore, M.M., Ahmad, A., Paul, A., Daniel, A.: Hadoop based real-time big data architecture for remote sensing earth observatory system. In: 2015 6th International Conference on Computing, Communication and Networking Technologies (ICCCNT), pp. 1–7 (2015)
6. Xhafa, F., Naranjo, V., Caball, S.: Processing and analytics of big data streams with Yahoo! S4. In: 2015 IEEE 29th International Conference on Advanced Information Networking and Applications, pp. 263–270 (2015)
7. Begum, S., Barua, S., Filla, R., Ahmed, M.U.: Classification of physiological signals for wheel loader operators using multi-scale entropy analysis and case-based reasoning. Expert Syst. Appl. **41**, 295–305 (2014)
8. Begum, S., Barua, S., Ahmed, M.U.: Physiological sensor signals classification for healthcare using sensor data fusion and case-based reasoning. Sensors **14**, 11770 (2014)

9. Barua, S., Begum, S., Ahmed, M.U.: Clustering based approach for automated EEG artifacts handling. In: 13th Scandinavian Conference on Artificial Intelligence (SCAI 2015) (2015)
10. Fu, T.-C.: A review on time series data mining. Eng. Appl. Artif. Intell. **24**, 164–181 (2011)
11. Ahmed, M.U., Funk, P.: A computer aided system for post-operative pain treatment combining knowledge discovery and case-based reasoning. In: Agudo, B.D., Watson, I. (eds.) ICCBR 2012. LNCS (LNAI), vol. 7466, pp. 3–16. Springer, Heidelberg (2012). https://doi.org/10.1007/978-3-642-32986-9_3
12. Banaee, H., Ahmed, M.U., Loutfi, A.: Data mining for wearable sensors in health monitoring systems: a review of recent trends and challenges. Sensors **13**, 17472–17500 (2013)
13. Ahmed, M.U., Banaee, H., Loutfi, A.: Health monitoring for elderly: an application using case-based reasoning and cluster analysis. ISRN Artif. Intell. **2013**, 11 (2013)
14. Arico, P., Borghini, G., Di Flumeri, G., Sciaraffa, N., Colosimo, A., Babiloni, F.: Passive BCI in operational environments: insights, recent advances and future trends. IEEE Trans. Biomed. Eng. **64**, 1431–1436 (2017)

Run-Time Assurance
for the E-care@home System

Mobyen Uddin Ahmed[1(✉)], Hossein Fotouhi[1], Uwe Köckemann[3],
Maria Lindén[1], Ivan Tomasic[1], Nicolas Tsiftes[2], and Thiemo Voigt[2]

[1] Mälardalen University, Västerås, Sweden
mobyen.ahmed@mdh.se
[2] RISE SICS, Stockholm, Sweden
[3] Örebro University, Örebro, Sweden

Abstract. This paper presents the design and implementation of the
software for a run-time assurance infrastructure in the E-care@home system. An experimental evaluation is conducted to verify that the run-time
assurance infrastructure is functioning correctly, and to enable detecting performance degradation in experimental IoT network deployments
within the context of E-care@home.

1 Introduction

Making IoT networks more dependable is critical in applications such as assisted
living facilities [1]. One way towards achieving this goal is to increase the visibility into the operation of the network to developers, researchers, and system
operators. In essence, it should be possible to quickly get warnings about issues
that require attention in order for the system to operate correctly and with
acceptable performance. Such issues can be, for example, when a node's Battery
Level (BL) is low, or when the network is experiencing high packet loss rates.
Another objective is that we wish to keep long-term records of the historical performance in various metrics for each IoT device to find anomalies and changes
in trends of system performance.

To this end, we present a software infrastructure for *Run-Time Assurance*
(RTA) in the E-care@home system [2]. We define *run-time assurance* as a service that continuously runs to discover and report system errors and performance problems. At a high level, one can summarize the core functionality of
the run-time assurance infrastructure as the following three actions: (a) monitor
a variety of internal and external operating conditions periodically, (b) analyze
the collected data to find current performance degradations, or changes in the
environment that might affect future performance, and (c) report important
information to a system operator.

The challenges of building an infrastructure for RTA are threefold. First,
we must identify which protocols and parameters to monitor, with low overlapping of data that describe the same condition. Second, the monitoring must
be conducted with low overhead and with minimum interruption of regular

© ICST Institute for Computer Sciences, Social Informatics and Telecommunications Engineering 2018
M. U. Ahmed et al. (Eds.): HealthyIoT 2017, LNICST 225, pp. 107–110, 2018.
https://doi.org/10.1007/978-3-319-76213-5_15

E-care@home application-layer data packets. Third, since the monitoring relies on a potentially faulty communication link to transmit the results, the RTA must comprise parallel monitoring efforts at the server-side.

Our run-time assurance infrastructure consists of four different components that address these challenges: (a) RTA for sensor platforms, (b) database storage of RTA information, (c) RTA at the server-side, and (d) a graphical user interface for RTA. Together, these components provide an RTA service for all parts of an e-health system, including static sensor nodes for environmental monitoring, mobile sensor nodes for health parameter monitoring, and the data collection server for the aforementioned sensor nodes.

2   Run-Time Assurance Infrastructure

The E-care@home system uses a database as a central point of storage for data collection from heterogeneous sources. The inclusion of a relational database in a remote monitoring system has been shown before not to introduce a significant latency in the system [3]. We extended the database for RTA data, including received and lost packets, timestamps between messages, as well as several statistics related to the IoT network protocols used in the E-care@home system (i.e., RPL and TSCH). Data is entered into the database from a server application that receives data from variety of sensors. We distinguish between RTA data collected on the client side and the server side.

The power consumption of a node can reveal insights as to whether it is operating correctly and efficiently. For E-care@home's environmental monitoring nodes, which use the Contiki OS, we rely on software-based power profiling [4], which provides visibility into the power consumption of various system components and software modules. We periodically measure the amount of time that (1) the radio has been in transmission mode (TX), (2) the radio has been in reception mode (RX), (3) the micro-controller has been in active mode (CPU), and (4) the micro-controller has been in Low Power Mode (LPM). The CPU time and the LPM time are both needed to calculate the percentage of time that the CPU is in active mode.

For medical health monitoring, we use Shimmer sensors that communicate using Bluetooth radio. Each Shimmer device has the ability to measure low-noise accelerometer, wide-range accelerometer, gyroscope, magnetometer, pressure, temperature, battery voltage, external expansion ADCs, and ECG/EMG. For our experiments with the RTA infrastructure, we collect sensor id, various physiological measurements, number of received packets, number of lost packets, BL (calculated at the Shimmer device), and local timestamps.

RTA packets are collected by the server together with regular sensor data packets. For the Contiki server software, we have a Python script that receives and parses messages from the IoT network's border router. For the Shimmer server software, we use Shimmer firmware, which is an application that can receive data from a Shimmer device using Bluetooth. This software acts as an API for the server-side to collect data. In order to get the raw values of BL together with medical parameters, we modified the firmware source code to be able to send these readings to an E-care@home database, where they can be obtained for analysis and presentation to a network operator.

At the server side, we are keeping track of the following metrics related to packet reception. The *signal strength* is collected to find if the radio environment of a node deteriorates. If the deteriorated condition persists over a long time, this may indicate that the physical topology of the network should be adjusted. The *Packet Reception Rate* (PRR) shows whether the application-layer packets get through from each sensor node to the gateway server. The PRR will be affected by the quality of the radio environment, network routing, traffic load, packet buffer space, and other system-level conditions. The *communication interruption time* is collected to warn when we have not received data from a specific node in a selected time period. The PRR is insufficient to warn about communication interruption because the PRR can take a long time to change significantly, depending on the time range for packet statistics that is used to calculate the PRR.

3   Evaluation

For brevity, we show only excerpts from our experimental evaluation of RTA within the E-care@home system, including both environmental and medical sensors. Figure 1 shows the radio duty cycles for nine Contiki nodes used for environmental monitoring. The TX duty cycle is on average below 0.5% across all nodes. The amount of time in the RX mode is below 2.5% on average. The data was collected by the RTA infrastructure over 1.68 days.

To evaluate the RTA of Shimmer devices, we deployed three sensors in three different rooms, where one of them was located closer to the destination (server). Two sensors sending measurements with 512 Hz, while having low BL (average of 1778 and 1801 mV) and one sending with 32 Hz with 3761 mV average BL. Figure 2 shows the PRR fluctuation over a period of around 12 h. There are some fluctuations at the beginning of the experiment, which are due to the existence of high environmental noise during the working hours. Shimmer 1 and Shimmer 2 with higher sampling frequency were depleted faster, resulting in some fluctuations at the end of the experiment, and eventually sudden PRR reductions.

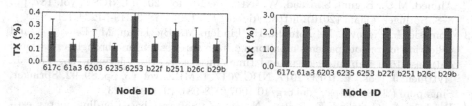

Fig. 1. TX (left) and RX (right) radio duty cycles for nine Contiki nodes. Note that the figures have different Y-axis scales.

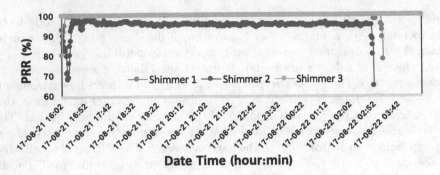

Fig. 2. Packet reception rates of three Shimmer sensors located in different rooms.

4 Conclusion

This paper describes the run-time assurance of the E-care@home system. We conducted an experimental evaluation that includes environmental sensor nodes running Contiki, and medical sensor nodes based on the Shimmer platform. We observed the packet reception rate and battery level in the Shimmer experiments. According to the experimental results, our RTA software shows the ability to monitor the PRR and battery level in real-time. Moreover, our evaluation with Contiki nodes shows that we can effectively collect important data for RTA while keeping the radio duty cycles at the same level as a system without an RTA service.

Acknowledgments. This work and the authors are supported by the distributed environment E-care@Home, funded by the Swedish Knowledge Foundation 2015–2019; and partially by the Embedded Sensor System for Health (ESS-H) research profile.

References

1. Fairbairn, M.L., Bate, I., Stankovic, J.: Improving the dependability of sensornets. In: Proceedings of Distributed Computing in Sensor Systems (DCOSS), Cambridge, Massachusetts, USA (2013)
2. Loutfi, A., Jönsson, A., Karlsson, L., Lind, L., Linden, M., Pecora, F., Voigt, T.: Ecare@Home: a distributed research environment on semantic interoperability. In: Ahmed, M.U., Begum, S., Raad, W. (eds.) HealthyIoT 2016. LNICST, vol. 187, pp. 3–8. Springer, Cham (2016). https://doi.org/10.1007/978-3-319-51234-1_1
3. Tomasic, I., Petrović, N., Fotouhi, H., Lindén, M., Björkman, M.: Data flow and collection for remote patients monitoring: from wireless sensors through a relational database to a web interface in real time. In: Eskola, H., Väisänen, O., Viik, J., Hyttinen, J. (eds.) EMBEC 2017, NBC 2017. IFMBE, vol. 65, pp. 89–92. Springer, Singapore (2018). https://doi.org/10.1007/978-981-10-5122-7_23
4. Dunkels, A., Österlind, F., Tsiftes, N., He, Z.: Software-based on-line energy estimation for sensor nodes. In: Proceedings of the IEEE Workshop on Embedded Networked Sensor Systems (IEEE Emnets), Cork, Ireland, June 2007

Scalable Framework for Distributed Case-Based Reasoning for Big Data Analytics

Shaibal Barua[✉] , Shahina Begum ,
and Mobyen Uddin Ahmed

School of Innovation, Design and Engineering, Mälardalen University,
721 23 Västerås, Sweden
{shaibal.barua, shahina.begum, mobyen.ahmed}@mdh.se

Abstract. This paper proposes a scalable framework for distributed case-based reasoning methodology to provide actionable knowledge based on historical big amount of data. The framework addresses several challenges, i.e., *promptly analyse big data, cross-domain, use-case specific data processing, multi-source case representation, dynamic case-management, uncertainty, check the plausibility of solution after adaptation* etc. through its' five modules architectures. The architecture allows the functionalities with distributed data analytics and intended to provide solutions under different conditions, i.e. data size, velocity, variety etc.

Keywords: Distributed analytics · Case-based reasoning

1 Introduction

The Internet-of-Things (IoT) paradigm is becoming key technologies for innovative products and applications. Smart objects can communicate and interact with each other in a defined IoT enabled environment and make autonomous decisions by appropriate correlation and association of data collected from the environment [1]. The envisioned I-IoT system senses the environment, and makes decision to sensed environmental changes dynamically and effectively with optimal resources, low cost and increased convenience. Such systems bring the following main generic research challenges:

- Heterogeneous data management that makes adequate and standard formats, models and sematic description of the data to support I-IoT systems in automated reasoning.
- Smart objects can autonomously respond to a wide range of circumstances without human interventions. Consequently, these systems must have the ability to reason efficiently about contextual information.
- These systems should interact with each other with the ability to operate distribute manner which is natural in IoT environment.
- Automated decision-making should be able to handle time critical situation and would provide fast and accurate decisions.

Today, the methodologies used for such systems are not particularly focused and are rather sparse. So, from system-level perspective, in implementation of such I-IoT

© ICST Institute for Computer Sciences, Social Informatics and Telecommunications Engineering 2018
M. U. Ahmed et al. (Eds.): HealthyIoT 2017, LNICST 225, pp. 111–114, 2018.
https://doi.org/10.1007/978-3-319-76213-5_16

systems, the current need is to investigate and determine core principles and algorithms. Case-based reasoning (CBR) is a methodology that solves a new problem by remembering and using previously solved problems that are similar to the current problem [2, 8, 10]. CBR can avoid the re-invent the wheel approach by remembering and using knowledge base. Moreover, sub-tasks of CBR such as case base maintenance, cases retrieval, cases adaptation and retaining new cases [3, 9] are well fitted for aforementioned challenges. However, currently there is no such distributed platform for CBR system that can meet the requirements of I-IoT and big data. Thus, this paper proposes both the state-of-the-art disciplinary and the system-oriented CBR architecture targeting to meet the generic research challenges. The proposed distributed CBR can be achieved through multi-agent CBR architecture, which can be beneficial for organizing knowledge base within the system and processing knowledge by the system [4] and maximum efficiency in I-IoT and Big data.

2   Related Work

Today even though IoT has generated excitement among the research community but still there are a number of challenges that need to be emphasized [5, 6]. An Intelligent IoT expects to exhibit intelligent behaviour by gathering multiple data and information, data management to avoid collusion, sensor fusion for robust decision, and cloud for information sharing and so on. In IoT, the gathered data needs to be managed with proper order and classification of data is also a vital part. In the field of IoT, a layer based data management system is presented in [5]. Due to globalization of IoT systems, it needs Cloud service for information sharing. A Cloud service for IoT architecture has been developed for Vehicular Data Cloud Services in [7]. Design of a generic scheme for I-IoT systems need to deal with several challenges and it needs to be able to handle the number of things and objects that will be connected in IoT contextual intelligence is crucial. Another issue is exchanging and analysing massive amount of data and the vast amount of data also need to be processed, and presented in a seamless, efficient and interpretable form.

3   Proposed Architecture

Figure 1 shows a system-oriented overview of the proposed scalable Framework for distributed case-based reasoning that illustrates the main conceptual components and their connections to each other. The overall architecture consists of five modules. The *first module* is the input sources from various smart devices and sensors connected through Internet. In this module data gathered from heterogeneous sources will be stored. As a scalable generic architecture, it is not sufficient to store only the data or signals but also to store application domain knowledge. The main objective in this module is pre-processing the gathered data, so the data is clean and noise free, and feature extraction. However, a multidisciplinary application should also include cross-domain and use case specific knowledge for future decision support.

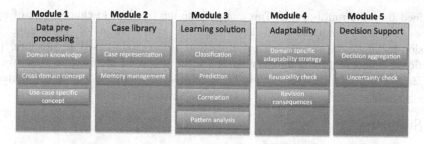

Fig. 1. Schematic diagram of the proposed case-based reasoning framework

To build a CBR system it requires to have a good knowledge base i.e., case libraries. An I-IoT system cannot be achievable without considering cloud environment. The *second module* creates collaborative case libraries in distributed manner for specific use cases and needs ability to reason efficiently about contextual information. Collaborative Big data management that makes adequate and standard formats, models and sematic description of the data using data and information processing and intelligent fusion algorithms, which will support I-IoT systems in automated reasoning. This will work with collaborative agent that can serve as the basis for automated systems that must collaborate with other local agents to interpret meaningful information from the data. One of the important modules is the *module 3* that performs various analytics for the CBR system. In the CBR, case retrieval is a major step, which seeks the most similar cases that corresponds to the target case. In the distributed multi-agent architecture, each CBR agent can be called to perform classification, prediction, and/or patterns analysis either on a single or multiple dataset. This will depend on how the case library is requested from the data storage and here one goal is to achieve the scalability through parallelism in cloud based environment.

Since knowledge bases are distributed across several nodes in clusters and a multidisciplinary application e.g., healthcare application often needs case adaption, hence *module 4* has design to perform domain specific adaptability strategy, uncertainty check in case adaption that ensures reusability of case in future learning and decision making. Last but not least, *module 5* needs to aggregate the results that are

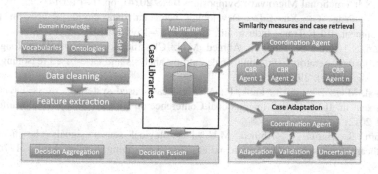

Fig. 2. Functional diagram of the proposed case-based reasoning framework

obtained from the multi-agents. This can provide the freedom to choose type of analytics i.e., using individualized knowledge or combination of knowledge for decision-making, and manage highest utilization of the cloud-based architecture. The functional connectivity among the modules in the proposed architecture is shown in Fig. 2. The functionalities should also be scalable depends of the application domain.

4 Summary

The IoT will be a basis for the future connected smart systems and sustainable infrastructures. Data management using IoT and Big data analysis on the cloud is going to be the most potential for a strong economic impact in the coming decades for the smart services. The paper has emphasized on the generic architecture for autonomous systems of future Intelligent Internet of Things (I-IoT). In addition, this system can be implemented on big data platform such as Spark with the existing support of distributed functionalities. Thus, cloud to connect intelligent things can be conducted by connecting sensors, data fusion and management through IoT; also apply them to big data analysis for automated decision-making by the scalable computing resources in the cloud.

References

1. Miorandi, D., Sicari, S., De Pellegrini, F., Chlamtac, I.: Internet of things: vision, applications and research challenges. Ad Hoc Netw. **10**(7), 1497–1516 (2012)
2. Kolodner, J.: An introduction to case-based reasoning. Artif. Intell. Rev. **6**(1), 3–34 (1992). (in English)
3. Aamodt, A., Plaza, E.: Case-based reasoning: foundational issues, methodological variations, and system approaches. AI Commun. **7**(1), 39–59 (1994)
4. Plaza, E., McGinty, L.: Distributed case-based reasoning. Knowl. Eng. Rev. **20**(3), 261–265 (2006)
5. Ma, M., Wang, P., Chu, C.H.: Data management for Internet of Things: challenges, approaches and opportunities. In: 2013 IEEE International Conference on Green Computing and Communications and IEEE Internet of Things and IEEE Cyber, Physical and Social Computing, pp. 1144–1151 (2013)
6. Jianguo, M.: Internet-of-Things: technology evolution and challenges. In: 2014 IEEE MTT-S International Microwave Symposium (IMS 2014), pp. 1–4 (2014)
7. He, W., Yan, G., Xu, L.D.: Developing vehicular data cloud services in the IoT environment. IEEE Trans. Industr. Inf. **10**(2), 1587–1595 (2014)
8. Begum, S., Barua, S., Filla, R., Ahmed, M.U.: Classification of physiological signals for wheel loader operators using multi-scale entropy analysis and case-based reasoning. Expert Syst. Appl. **41**(2), 295–305 (2014)
9. Ahmed, M.U., Begum, S., Funk, P.: A hybrid case-based system in stress diagnosis and treatment. In: IEEE-EMBS International Conference on Biomedical and Health Informatics (BHI 2012) (2012)
10. Begum, S., Barua, S., Ahmed, M.U.: Physiological sensor signals classification for healthcare using sensor data fusion and case-based reasoning. Sensors **14**(7), 11770–11785 (2014)

Deep Learning Based Person Identification Using Facial Images

Hamidur Rahman[✉], Mobyen Uddin Ahmed, and Shahina Begum

School of Innovation, Design and Engineering, Mälardalen University,
72123 Västerås, Sweden
{hamidur.rahman,mobyenUddin.ahmed,
shahina.begum}@mdh.se

Abstract. Person identification is an important task for many applications for example in security. A person can be identified using finger print, vocal sound, facial image or even by DNA test. However, Person identification using facial images is one of the most popular technique which is non-contact and easy to implement and a research hotspot in the field of pattern recognition and machine vision. In this paper, a deep learning based Person identification system is proposed using facial images which shows higher accuracy than another traditional machine learning, i.e. Support Vector Machine.

Keywords: Face recognition · Person identification · Deep learning

1 Introduction

Person identification using facial images is one of the most popular biometric topics in computer vision community because of its broad applications such as human-computer interaction (HCI), homeland security, entertainment etc. Identifying a person using their facial images includes image processing and a classification based on machine learning can be defined as face recognition. However, this still remains a challenging problem because of intra-subject variations due to head pose, illumination, facial expression, occlusion due to the person themselves, other objects or accessories, facial hair, aging and so on [1].

A facial recognition technique is proposed by Chennamma et al. using SIFT features [2] where frontal facial images are used for training and manipulated facial images are used for testing. Even though the method shows higher accuracy than popular eigen face approach, the method is slower due to searching large number of matching points. Another novel face recognition algorithm method based on adaptive 3-D Local Binary Pattern and Singular Value Decomposition method is proposed in [3]. The experimental simulation results show good feature extraction effect and face recognition performance comparing other state-of-the-art methodologies. Another facial recognition method is proposed using generalized mean deep learning neural network [4]. The algorithm provides fast convergence of the feature set and the performance of the proposed algorithm is better in terms of identification accuracy. Deep learning models achieve higher accuracy in the field of object detection, text classification, image classification,

© ICST Institute for Computer Sciences, Social Informatics and Telecommunications Engineering 2018
M. U. Ahmed et al. (Eds.): HealthyIoT 2017, LNICST 225, pp. 115–119, 2018.
https://doi.org/10.1007/978-3-319-76213-5_17

facial recognition, gender classification, scene-classification, digits and traffic signs recognition etc. where it uses large architectures with numerous features [5].

In this paper, a person identification system using facial images i.e. facial recognition using deep learning is proposed. A deep learning model called Alexnet [6] is used for facial recognition which has 23 layers including five convolution layers, max-pooling layers, dropout layers and three fully connected layers. Alexnet is a specific type of deep learning algorithm that can both perform classification and extract features from raw images.

2 Materials and Methods

2.1 Data Collection

For this experiment both a public online image database and local image database (i.e. created internally by us) are used. Online public database AT&T[1] is a widely used face database for face recognition problem. The database has 400 gray scale images of 40 distinct subjects each for 10 different images. For some subjects, the images are captured at different situations such as times, lighting, facial expressions etc. All the images are captured against a dark homogeneous background with the subjects in an upright, frontal position. Images are saved in PGM format and the size of each image is 92×112 pixels, with 256 grey levels per pixel. Another image database called 'IDT' containing 50 color images of five subject is created locally by us. Ten different color images of different face angle are captured for each subject and saved all the images in JPG format in the 'IDT' database. In this database, each image size is 640×480 though later image size is changed into 227×227 pixels. During this data collection, environmental illumination is not constant and background is also not homogeneous.

2.2 Methods

In this paper work, facial recognition is performed using both traditional machine learning algorithm i.e. Support Vector Machine (SVM) and deep learning algorithm which are later compared for evaluation. Using both the databases 70% of the images are randomly selected for training and 30% of the images are selected for testing. In machine learning approach, i.e. SVM, HOG (Histogram of Oriented Gradients) features are extracted using MATLAB function 'extractHOGFeatures' [7] both for training and test images. For example, SVM is used in other domain such as stress classification [8] or physical activity classification [9]. To build a model, supervised machine learning model i.e. multiclass Support Vector Machine (SVM) [10] is used which is actually $K*(K-1)/2$ binary SVM model where K is the number of unique class labels. In the model one-versus-one coding design are considered and linear kernel function (i.e. dot product) is used. To identify an input image using the learned model, first face detection is performed using Viola-and-Jones algorithm [11] and HOG features are

---

[1] "AT&T Face Database: http://www.cl.cam.ac.uk/research/dtg/attarchive/facedatabase.html."

extracted from the registered facial image. SVM classifier is used for matching database feature vector with query feature vector. It finds best matching faces from the database and gives ID of best matching face image as a recognition output. An overview of the model is presented in Fig. 1.

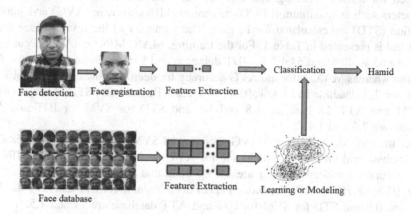

Face detection   Face registration   Feature Extraction   Classification   Hamid

Face database   Feature Extraction   Learning or Modeling

Fig. 1. Face recognition overview

Deep learning algorithms can learn features, representations, and tasks directly from images which eliminate the hassle of manual feature selection. In this study, a deep learning model called Alexnet [6] is used. Alexnet has 25 layers including one input layers, five convolution layers, seven Relu (Rectified Linear Unit) layers, three maximum pooling layers, two cross channel normalization layers, two dropout layers, three fully connected layers, one softmax layer and one output layers. Since Alexnet network was trained on 227×227-pixel images, all of our images are resized into the same resolution. The first layer of the Alexnet is input layer where the resolution of the images is assigned which are $227 \times 227 \times 3$ and 227×227 for IDT and ATT database respectively. The last layer is output layer which uses probabilities returned by softmax activation function for each input to assign it to one of the mutually exclusive classes. An overview of deep learning based facial recognition is presented in Fig. 2.

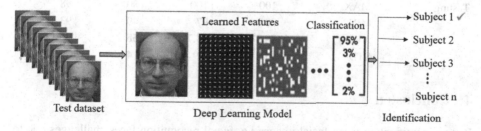

Test dataset   Learned Features   Classification   Subject 1 ✓
    Subject 2
    95%
    3%   Subject 3
    ⋮
    2%   Subject n
Deep Learning Model   Identification

Fig. 2. Deep learning face recognition

3 Results and Evaluation

Both SVM and deep learning (DL) approaches are run 10 times for both the database. Every time a random 70% of the images are used for training and the rest of the images are used for testing. Training and test accuracy are calculated and then statistical parameters such as maximum (MAX), minimum (MIN), average (AVG) and standard deviation (STD) are calculated for 10 runs. The summary of the result of face recognition test is presented in Table 1. For the training, MAX, MIN and AVG accuracy of SVM are 65%, 40% and 54.4% for IDT database and 91%, 86% and 88.8% for ATT database whereas MAX, MIN and AVG accuracy for deep learning are 100%, 94% and 96.2% for IDT database and 100%, 95%, 98% for ATT database. STD of deep learning for IDT and ATT database are 1.8 and 1.6 and STD for SVM for IDT and ATT database are 7.6 and 1.4.

For the test, MAX, MIN and AVG accuracy of SVM are 80%, 40% and 58% for IDT database and 98%, 93% and 95.1% for ATT database whereas MAX, MIN and AVG accuracy for deep learning are 100%, 80% and 88.3% for IDT database and 100%, 97%, 98.7% for ATT database. STD of deep learning for IDT and ATT database are 6 and 0.9 and STD for SVM for IDT and ATT database are 14 and 1.5.

It is observed that traditional machine learning algorithm, i.e. SVM does not work well when images are not captured in controlled environment (i.e. homogeneous background constant illumination, equal distance between camera and face etc.) while DL algorithm works better for any kind of images because of its rich feature extraction capability. STD of DL and SVM are 0.9 and 1.5 for ATT database and 6 and 14 for IDT database which indicates that the fluctuation of accuracy for each run for ATT database is less than IDT database due to higher number of data sets.

Table 1. Statistical measurement of face recognition accuracy

Training/Testing	Statistical parameters	DL accuracy		SVM accuracy	
		IDT database	ATT database	IDT database	ATT database
Training	MAX	100	100	65	91
	MIN	94	95	40	86
	AVG	**96.2**	**98**	**54.4**	**88.8**
	STD	1.83	1.6	7.6	1.4
Testing	MAX	100	100	80	98
	MIN	80	97	40	93
	AVG	**88.3**	**98.7**	**58**	**95.1**
	STD	6.0	0.9	14	1.5

4 Conclusion

Person identification using facial images i.e. facial recognition faces challenges due to several complex situations such as intra-subject variations due to head pose, illumination, facial expression, occlusion due to other objects or accessories, facial hair, aging and so on. Both the traditional machine learning algorithm i.e. SVM and deep learning algorithm are used for facial recognition and results show that deep learning based approach provide higher accuracy level than traditional machine learning approach. Results can be improved using larger dataset for better training model in internal database. A real time facial recognition using deep learning is considered as future work.

Acknowledgement. The authors would like to acknowledge the Swedish Knowledge Foundation (KKS), Hök instrument AB, Volvo Car Corporation (VCC), The Swedish National Road and Transport Research Institute (VTI), Autoliv AB, Prevas AB Sweden, and all the test subjects for their support of the research projects in this area.

References

1. Olszewska, J.I.: Automated face recognition: challenges and solutions. In: Ramakrishnan, S. (ed.) Pattern Recognition - Analysis and Applications, Chap. 4. InTech, Rijeka (2016)
2. Chennamma, H.R., Rangarajan, L., Veerabhadrappa: Face identification from manipulated facial images using SIFT. In: 2010 3rd International Conference on Emerging Trends in Engineering and Technology, pp. 192–195 (2010)
3. Li, Y.: Novel face recognition algorithm based on adaptive 3D local binary pattern features and improved Singular Value Decomposition method. In: 2016 International Conference on Inventive Computation Technologies (ICICT), pp. 1–7 (2016)
4. Sharma, P., Yadav, R.N., Arya, K.V.: Face recognition from video using generalized mean deep learning neural network. In: 2016 4th International Symposium on Computational and Business Intelligence (ISCBI), pp. 195–199 (2016)
5. Islam, S.M.S., Rahman, S., Rahman, M.M., Dey, E.K., Shoyaib, M.: Application of deep learning to computer vision: a comprehensive study. In: 2016 5th International Conference on Informatics, Electronics and Vision (ICIEV), pp. 592–597 (2016)
6. Krizhevsky, A., Sutskever, I., Hinton, G.E.: ImageNet classification with deep convolutional neural networks. In: Advances in Neural Information Processing Systems (2012)
7. Dalal, N., Triggs, B.: Histograms of oriented gradients for human detection. In: 2005 IEEE Computer Society Conference on Computer Vision and Pattern Recognition (CVPR 2005), vol. 1, pp. 886–893 (2005)
8. Barua, S., Begum, S., Ahmed, M.U.: Supervised machine learning algorithms to diagnose stress for vehicle drivers based on physiological sensor signals. In: 12th International Conference on Wearable Micro and Nano Technologies for Personalized Health (2015)
9. Ahmed, M.U., Loutfi, A.: Physical activity identification using supervised machine learning and based on pulse rate. Int. J. Adv. Comput. Sci. Appl. (IJACSA) 4(7), 209 (2013)
10. Rajesh, K.M., Naveenkumar, M.: A robust method for face recognition and face emotion detection system using support vector machines. In: 2016 International Conference on Electrical, Electronics, Communication, Computer and Optimization Techniques (ICEEC-COT), pp. 1–5 (2016)
11. Viola, P., Jones, M.: Robust real-time face detection. In: Proceedings, Eighth IEEE International Conference on Computer Vision, ICCV 2001, p. 747 (2001)

Erratum to: Internet of Things (IoT) Technologies for HealthCare

Mobyen Uddin Ahmed, Shahina Begum, and Jean-Baptiste Fasquel

Erratum to:
M. U. Ahmed et al. (Eds.):
Internet of Things (IoT) Technologies for HealthCare, **LNICST 225,**
https://doi.org/10.1007/978-3-319-76213-5

In an older version of this proceedings volume, there was a mistake in the third editor Name. This has now been corrected

---

The updated online version of this book can be found at
https://doi.org/10.1007/978-3-319-76213-5

© ICST Institute for Computer Sciences, Social Informatics and Telecommunications Engineering 2018
M. U. Ahmed et al. (Eds.): HealthyIoT 2017, LNICST 225, p. E1, 2018.
https://doi.org/10.1007/978-3-319-76213-5_18

Author Index

Abraham, Pierre   42
Ahmed, Mobyen Uddin   10, 26, 101, 107, 111, 115
Alrashed, Muntadar   54
Ambourg, Alexandre   3

Barua, Shaibal   26, 111
Begum, Shahina   10, 26, 101, 111, 115
Björkman, Mats   48
Bosche, Jerome   75

Carette, Romuald   75
Catalina, Carlos Alberto   101
Chauvet, Pierre   82
Cilia, Federica   75
Collette, Mathieu   69

Daya, Bassam   82
Dequen, Gilles   75
Di Flumeri, Gianluca   101

Ebert, André   62

Fasquel, Jean-Baptiste   42
Fotouhi, Hossein   48, 107
Frindel, Carole   3, 19

Gard, Pierre   3
Gardašević, Gordana   48
Gibaud, Marc   82
Guerin, Jean-Luc   75

Hassine, Naoures   69
Henni, Samir   42
Hök, Bertil   101
Humeau-Heurtier, Anne   42

Jamin, Antoine   42
Jrad, Nisrine   82

Köckemann, Uwe   107

Lalanne, Lucie   3
Le Bouquin Jeannès, R.   34
Leftheriotis, Georges   42, 69
Lesueur, François   3
Limonad, Lior   101
Lindén, Maria   48, 107
Linnhoff-Popien, Claudia   62

Marouane, Chadly   62

Nguyen The Tich, Sylvie   82
Nguyen, L. P.   34

Palombo, Carlo   69

Raad, Muhammad Wasim   54
Rahman, Hamidur   10, 115
Rousseau, David   3, 19

Saleh, M.   34
Saravanan, M.   88
Schang, Daniel   82
Schmid, Kyrill   62
Sheltami, Tarek   54
Shubha, R.   88
Soliman, Mohamed Abdelmonem   54

Tomasic, Ivan   48, 107
Tsiftes, Nicolas   107

Vahabi, Maryam   48
Vandromme, Luc   75
Voigt, Thiemo   107

Printed in the United States
by Bookmasters

Printed in the United States
By Bookmasters